The CYCLIST'S F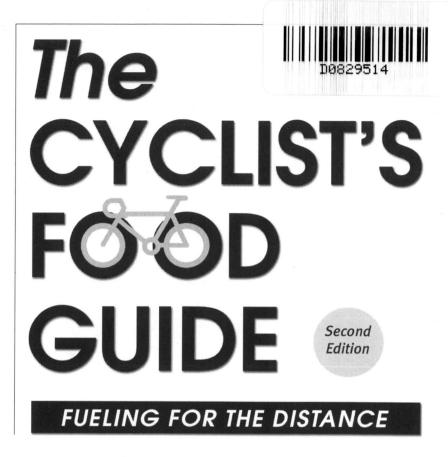D GUIDE

Second Edition

FUELING FOR THE DISTANCE

Nancy Clark, MS, RD
Jenny Hegmann, MS, RD

Foreword by Michael McCoy
Adventure Cycling Association

Sports Nutrition Publishers
West Newton, MA

Clark, Nancy 1951- Hegmann, Jenny 1965-
    The Cyclist's Food Guide: Fueling for the Distance, 2nd ed.
    p. cm
    Includes bibliographical references and index.
    LCCN 2004107717
    ISBN 0-9718911-2-8

    1. Sports—Nutrition 2. Bicycle riding
    I. Title

Complete Cataloging-in-Publication Data available on request

Book design by Patricia Robinson, Waban, MA, patrobinsondesign@mac.com

Cover photo: Mark Wojahn

Published in West Newton, MA, by Sports Nutrition Publishers
60 Lindbergh Avenue Suite 2A, West Newton, MA 02465
617-795-1875   sportsnutrition@rcn.com

This book is available at special discounts for bulk purchase. Special editions or book excerpts can also be created to specification. For details, contact the sales manager at Sports Nutrition Publishers.

Printed in the United States of America 10 9 8 7 6 5 4 3 2 1

The information contained in this book is not intended to serve as a substitute for professional medical advice. The authors and publisher specifically disclaim any and all liability arising directly or indirectly from the use of any information contained in this book. A health care professional should be consulted regarding your specific medical and nutritional concerns.
The web addresses cited were current as of May 2011.

We dedicate this book to the cyclists who give
of their time and energy to raise money for important
causes and help make the world a better place.
We want to help these everyday champions to eat
effectively, so they can enjoy high energy,
good health, and miles of enjoyable cycling.

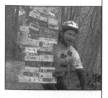

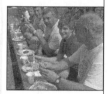

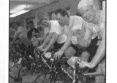

ACKNOWLEDGMENTS

FIRST OF ALL, WE OFFER ABUNDANT THANKS TO ADVENTURE CYCLING ASSOCIATION for their generosity in providing many of the photographs in this book and for their whole-hearted support for this project. Particular thanks goes to Greg Siple and Mike McCoy.

We appreciate the help from scores of cyclists all over the world—the randonneurs, cyclo-tourists, mountain bikers, racers, and recreational riders—who eagerly shared their personal food stories and nutrition tips.

We send our personal thanks to—
- Our loving families for their enthusiastic and supportive cheers.
- Paul, Jenny's chief support-crew, for his unfailing encouragement.
- Patricia Robinson, graphic designer, for creating a pleasing book from our words.
- John McGrath, Nancy's husband and business partner, for his publishing skills, wisdom, and never-ending support.
- The many cyclists near and far who have helped us understand their nutrition concerns, especially John Hughes, cycling coach and former Managing Director of the UltraMarathon Cycling Association, Adam Myerson of Cycle-Smart, Inc., Ed Kross, MaryAnn Martinez, the Northeast Bicycle Club, and Jessica Truslow. Their experiences help us to better help other cyclists win with nutrition.
- The cyclists who generously contributed their photos: Caroline Cardiasmenos (Rooted Tree Photography), Marcia Dana, Peter Doran (pdoranphoto.com), J. D. Hale and The Rippers, Mark McMaster, Vicki Samolyk, Aaldrik Tiktak, and Mark Wojahn.

And finally, we are indebted to the many cycling organizations and individuals whose love of biking has inspired them to educate and advocate for safe, fun, and accessible riding.

W HEN MY FUTURE WIFE NANCY AND I BEGAN PREPARING FOR OUR FIRST LONG-distance bicycle tour in 1974, we knew approximately as much about nutrition as we did about training for an epic tour. Which is to say, almost nothing (consider that our on-bike preparation for the cross-country trip consisted of a single 30-mile ride).

We had begun planning our summer ride while still snow-bound at Grand Targhee Ski Resort in the Wyoming Tetons, where Nancy and I had serendipitously met. In truth, I probably should have known something about nutrition, because my job at the resort was that of head night cook. However, the only items on the menu that I had to prepare were grilled steaks, baked potatoes, deep-fried shrimp and chicken, and tossed salad. And prior to that, my culinary experience boiled down to having once baking cherry cobbler in a Dutch oven for a Boy Scout merit badge.

Consequently, what ended up fueling us for the majority of the miles we pedaled between Seattle and Rhinelander, Wisconsin, was peanut butter, bread, peanut butter, Coca-Cola, and more peanut butter. When you're young, naturally energetic, and don't know any better, you seem to get away with eating just about anything and do fine. However, I'm sure we would've done even better had we eaten properly, which we no doubt would have, had a book like *The Cyclist's Food Guide* been available to us at the time.

Whether training, racing, riding for fitness, or touring, every cyclist can benefit from a well-considered nutritional program. Keeping your fuel level up is important, obviously, but so too is the relative octane of the fuel you put in your tank. I've found, in my experience as a road and mountain biker, 2:42 marathon runner, and Nordic skiing competitor, eating the right foods after exercise can speed up recovery, especially for master and senior athletes. And you can't find any better advice on how to go about obtaining optimal nutrition than you'll glean by reading Nancy Clark and Jenny Hegmann's *The Cyclist's Food Guide.*

Nancy Clark RD is an internationally known sports nutritionist, a dedicated bike commuter, and a 1978 TransAmerica tour leader. Her popular column The *Cyclist's Kitchen* is published in our association magazine, *Adventure Cyclist*, and she is also a regular contributor to *American Fitness* and active.com. Nancy has counseled an array of athletes, ranging from novice cyclists to members of the Boston Celtics and Red Sox. Jenny Hegmann RD, a registered dietitian specializing in sports nutrition, wellness, and weight management, is equally knowledgeable and passionate about providing nutritional advice for cyclists. She is a contributor for *UltraCycling* magazine. Rarely a day goes by that Jenny is not on her bike. She commutes to work and has participated in randonnées, fitness rides, and races.

Nancy and Jenny insightfully impart their common-sense information on preventing fatigue during long rides, controlling winter weight gain, and ensuring proper protein intake on a vegetarian diet—and these are just a few tastes of what you'll find in *The Cyclist's Food Guide*. A cornucopia of information, the book brims with dietary details that are easy to understand and incorporate into your everyday life. You'll get more out of your cycling—be it fitness riding, racing, touring, even indoor spinning—by absorbing and adopting the sound basics contained within this book.

We are blessed at Adventure Cycling to have the opportunity to meet hundreds of fascinating bicyclists during their cross-country tours. They commonly talk about food, whether their journeys are powered primarily by gummy bears and potato chips or by more nutritious fare. Through stressing the hows and whys of eating right, *The Cyclist's Food Guide* contains the ingredients necessary to get these and all riders onto the road to high energy, good health, and smooth cycling.

—Michael McCoy

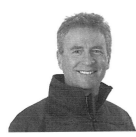

Michael McCoy has been involved with the Adventure Cycling Association (www.adventurecycling.org) since the organization began as Bikecentennial in the mid-1970s. Today he serves as field editor and staff writer, working from his home in Teton Valley, Idaho. His job is to help inspire people of all ages to travel by bicycle for fitness, fun, and self-discovery. Headquartered in Missoula, Montana, Adventure Cycling Association boasts 45,000 members, and its Adventure Cycling Route Network encompasses 40,700 miles of roads perfectly suited for cycling.

PHOTO COURTESY RU OUTSIDE

JENNY AND I HAVE COVERED MANY MILES ON OUR BIKES THROUGHOUT the years—commutes to work, century rides, transAmerica tours, randonnées, and races. As sports nutritionists, we have the advantage of knowing how to fuel our bodies for going and enjoying the distance.

Through our writing, counseling, and seminars, we have helped scores of active people achieve their goals with good nutrition. In this *Cyclist's Food Guide*, we combine our expertise in sports nutrition with our knowledge of cycling to deliver information that tells you how, what, and when to eat for optimal fueling and top performance.

Whether you are embarking on your first cycling adventure, your tenth tour, or your 100th race, we hope you will benefit from our practical, tried-and-true, and helpful advice. We provide ideas for easy meals, lists of foods, fluids, and nutrients, and tips from both coaches and experienced cyclists. Novice riders will find the words of wisdom they need to allay fears about running out of steam on the long rides and bonking on the hills. Seasoned riders, racers, and ultra-distance riders will find insight into sports supplements, timing of pre- and post-ride meals to enhance performance, and eating well despite long hours in the saddle.

When you put the information in *The Cyclist's Food Guide* into practice, you'll gain an edge over your peers who fuel their muscles poorly and fail to care for their health with premium nutrition.

We hope you make *The Cyclist's Food Guide* an integral part of your training program. It will answer your questions about nutrition for cycling, give you inspiration for the miles ahead, and help you fuel the distance strongly, whatever your cycling goals.

With best wishes for safe, smooth, and successful riding,

—*Nancy Clark, MS, RD, CSSD and Jenny Hegmann, MS, RD*

The CYCLIST'S F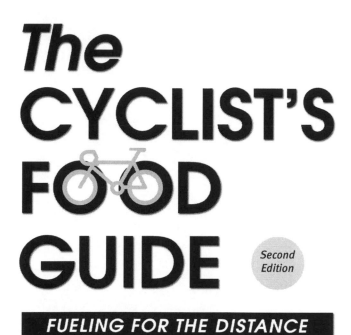OD GUIDE

Second Edition

FUELING FOR THE DISTANCE

CHAPTER 1

Your Daily Diet: Eating for Health and High Energy

"I've got my training down, but nutrition is my missing link."

TOO MANY CYCLISTS OF ALL AGES AND ABILITIES EXPRESS THIS CONCERN to us. They are frustrated with their low energy, inability to lose weight, and confusion about what to eat for an effective sports diet. Due to the time constraints that riding imposes upon already busy schedules, nutrition can easily become a missing link, particularly if you fail to plan for proper meals. This chapter reviews the basics of good nutrition for cyclists and will give you tips to make wise food decisions. Chapters 2 and 3 will give you ideas for quick and healthy breakfast, lunch, and dinner meals.

What is an effective sports diet? Whether you are at home, away, or on a tour, eating effectively means enjoying at least:
1. Three different kinds of food at each meal;
2. Two different kinds of food at each snack;
3. Evenly sized meals every four hours throughout the day (not "crescendo eating" with a small breakfast and lunch, followed by a large meal at the end of the day);
4. Ninety percent of the calories from quality foods and, if desired, the remaining 10 percent from sweets and treats.

Luckily for most of today's cyclists, you don't have to be a good cook to eat well. You can optimally nourish your body even if you are eating on the run and spending little time in the kitchen.

● DIETARY RECOMMENDATIONS FOR GOOD HEALTH

Before you eat, think about what goes into your mouth. Foods like vegetables, fruits, whole grains, low-fat dairy products, and lean protein foods contain the nutrients you need for health and performance. These guidelines from the U.S. Department of Agriculture's Center for Nutrition Policy and Promotion will help you choose an optimal sports diet.

Enjoy generous amounts of fruits and vegetables at every meal and snack.
- Eat red, orange, and dark green vegetables, such as tomatoes, sweet potatoes, and broccoli, in main and side dishes.
- Eat fruit, vegetables, or unsalted nuts as snacks—they are nature's original fast foods.

Switch to skim or 1% milk.
- They have the same amount of calcium and other essential nutrients as whole milk, but less fat and calories.
- Try calcium-fortified soy products as an alternative to dairy foods.

Make at least half your grains whole.
- Choose 100% whole-grain cereals, breads, crackers, rice, and pasta.
- Check the ingredients list on food packages to find whole-grain foods.

Vary your protein food choices.
- Twice a week, enjoy seafood for the protein on your plate.
- Eat beans, which are a natural source of fiber and protein.
- Keep meat and poultry portions small and lean.

Limit your intake of saturated fats.
- Major sources of saturated fats include cakes, cookies, ice cream, pizza, cheese, sausages, pepperoni, and greasy meat. Make them occasional choices.
- Select lean cuts of meats or poultry and fat-free or low-fat milk, yogurt, and cheese.

Switch from solid fats to oils when preparing food.
- Choose fewer foods with solid fats:
  - Beef, pork, and chicken fat
  - Butter, cream, and milk fat
  - Coconut, palm, and palm kernel oils

- Hydrogenated and partially hydrogenated oils
- Stick margarine and shortening
• Replace solid fats with vegetable oils when cooking:
- Canola, corn, cottonseed, olive, peanut, safflower
  and sunflower oils
- Tub (soft) margarine

Choose foods and drinks with little or no added sugars.
• When a sugar is close to first on the ingredients list, the food is high in added sugars. Some names for added sugars include sucrose, glucose, high fructose corn syrup, corn syrup, maple syrup, and fructose.
• Drink water instead of sugary drinks. There are about 10 packets of sugar in a 12-ounce can of soda and about 5 packets of sugar in 12 ounces of a sports drink. Save the sports drinks for during extended exercise!
• Select fruit for dessert. Eat sugary desserts less often.
• Choose 100% fruit juice instead of fruit-flavored drinks.

For more information and a link to a Food Tracker, visit www.ChooseMyPlate.gov.

Here are some guidelines to help you make optimal food choices:
• Eat lots of fruits and vegetables: a generous portion of fruit and/or vegetables at each meal and snack.
• Choose a variety of colors of fruits and vegetables each day: red apples, green peppers, orange carrots, white potatoes. Different colors offer different vitamins, minerals, and health-protective compounds.
• Enjoy whole-grain products at least two times per day, such as oatmeal for breakfast and whole-wheat bread for lunch. If you end up eating refined grains at some of your meals, they are not "worthless." Most refined grains, such as breads, pasta, and cereals, are enriched with B-vitamins and iron, nutrients that are important for athletes. In general, at least half your grains should come from whole grains, which offer more fiber, trace minerals, and health protection. Whole grains include whole wheat, brown rice, oats, corn, and barley.

Food can be divided into five groups: grain, fruit, vegetable, milk (or calcium-rich food), and protein. The trick to balancing the recommended servings of foods during your day is to plan to have at least three out of five food groups per meal, and two or three food groups per snack, such as:

	Grain	Fruit	Vegetable	Milk	Protein
Breakfast:	bran flakes	banana	-----	milk	almonds
Lunch:	bread	apple	baby carrots	-----	tuna fish
Snack:	granola	berries	-----	yogurt	-----
Dinner:	spaghetti	-----	tomato sauce	Parmesan cheese	ground turkey
Snack:	popcorn	cider	-----	-----	-----

- Include a calcium-rich food at each meal. This could be milk (or calcium-fortified soymilk) on cereal, yogurt with lunch, a latte in the afternoon, and a pile of broccoli with dinner.
- When selecting and preparing meat, poultry, and milk or milk products, make choices that are lean, low-fat, or fat-free.
- Include a little healthy fat at each meal, but limit your intake of unhealthy saturated and trans fats. Healthy fats include olive and canola oils, nuts and nut butters, avocado, and oily fish such as salmon.

● **CARBOHYDRATES FOR YOUR SPORTS DIET**—By eating carbo-hydrate-rich fruits, vegetables, and grains as the foundation of each meal, you'll consume 55 to 65 percent of your calories from carbohydrates. This is exactly what you need for a high-energy sports diet. Carbohydrates are stored in muscles in the form of glycogen, the energy you need to train hard day after day, ride long distances, and compete well on race day.

Some cyclists believe they will get fat if they eat carbohy-drates such as breads, cereals, and pastas at each meal. False. Carbohydrates are not fattening; excess calories are fattening. (See chapter 16 for information on how to lose body fat.)

Fruits and Vegetables—Fruits and vegetables are excellent sources of carbohydrates that help to fuel your muscles. In addition, they are like nature's vitamin pills, providing vitamin

Cyclists need not spend hours in the kitchen to have a healthful diet. The following foods offer top-quality nutrition and require little or no cooking.

Fruits

Citrus fruits and brightly colored fruits have the most nutrients. The following are rich in beta-carotene and/or vitamin C:

- Oranges
- Grapefruit
- Clementines
- Cantaloupe
- Strawberries
- Mango
- Kiwi
- Dried apricots

Vegetables

Dark green leafy, orange-fleshed, and brightly colored vegetables have the most nutrients. Here are some good sources of beta-carotene and/or vitamin C:

- Broccoli
- Spinach, romaine and other dark green lettuce
- Green, red, and yellow peppers
- Tomatoes, fresh, canned, or sun-dried
- Carrots
- Sweet potato
- Winter squash

Milk

Milk products offer a naturally good source of calcium and include:

- Milk or flavored milk, preferably low-fat or fat-free
- Yogurt, preferably low-fat or fat-free
- Cheese, preferably reduced-fat

Non-milk sources of calcium include:

- Calcium-fortified orange juice, soymilk, and tofu

Meat and other protein

Healthful proteins that are fast and simple include:

- Canned tuna and salmon
- Hummus
- Canned beans: black, pinto, kidney, refried beans
- Nuts and nut butters: peanut, sunflower, almond
- Deli roast beef, ham, and turkey; rotisserie chicken
- Tofu
- Roasted soynuts
- Cottage cheese

Grains

Cook-free grains offer carbohydrates, B-vitamins, and fiber:

- High-fiber or whole-grain breakfast cereals (preferably iron-enriched)
- Low-fat granola or meusli
- Wholesome breads, rolls, and bagels
- Whole-wheat pita pockets, sandwich wraps, and tortillas
- Whole-grain crackers

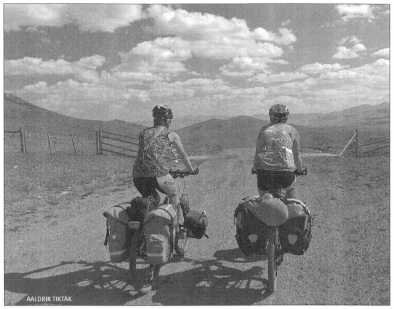

The food choices you make today will affect your performance, health, and ability to enjoy riding in the years to come, so choose wisely. Routinely eat healthful meals abundant with whole grains, fruits, and vegetables.

C, beta-carotene, fiber, and many other natural compounds that help maintain health and prevent disease. Research has repeatedly shown that diets rich in fruits and vegetables are protective against cancer, heart disease, and many other chronic health problems. But eating the minimum recommendation of 2 cups of fruit and 2½ cups of vegetables each day is another story. As one cyclist remarked, "I'm lucky if I eat that much in a week!" The trick is to eat large portions of them and to try to sneak them into your diet wherever possible—fruit in your morning cereal, dried fruit during a ride, or extra veggies in your lunchtime sandwich.

Tips to Boost Your Fruit Intake

The recommended daily intake for fruits is 2 cups or more a day. Here's what counts as 1 cup:

Orange juice	8 ounces	240 ml
Apple	1 small	100 g
Banana	1 small	100 g
Canned fruit	1 cup	240 g
Dried fruit	½ cup	80 g

Hungry cyclists can easily consume double portions and achieve the recommended intake.

The following tips may help you to increase your fruit intake:

- Enjoy a fruit smoothie for breakfast: blend together orange juice, a banana, frozen berries, some yogurt or protein powder, and whatever else sounds good to you.
- Top hot or cold breakfast cereal with extra sliced banana, blueberries, and strawberries.
- Keep fresh fruit in plain sight on the kitchen table, ready to grab and go.
- Keep cut-up melon, washed strawberries, peeled orange sections, and other fruits in the refrigerator. Store them in easy-to-open containers, and have toothpicks handy to help you snack right out of the fridge.
- Make little snack-baggies with dried fruit, like pineapple, apricots, figs, and dates, and enjoy them in place of sports candies while you bike.
- Keep canned and frozen fruits on hand, so when you run out of fresh fruit, you have an option.
- Add mandarin oranges, dried cranberries, or grapes to a salad.
- Snack on banana or apple slices with peanut butter.
- Enjoy frozen fruit bars as a post-ride refresher.

Tips to Boost Your Vegetable Intake

The recommended daily amount for vegetables is 2½ cups or more each day. Here's what counts as 1 cup:

Broccoli	1 medium stalk	200 g
Spinach	2 cups raw	60 g
Salad bar	1 average bowl	100 g
Spaghetti sauce (tomato)	1 cup	250 g

You may wish to eat double portions to help you meet the recommended amount. But if you still find it a struggle to eat enough veggies, the following tips may help enhance your vegetable intake, and your health:

- Eat more of the best vegetables, less of the rest. In general, colorful dark green, deep yellow, orange, and red vegetables have far more nutrients than pale ones. Hence, if you dislike pale zucchini, summer squash, and cucumbers, don't work hard to acquire a taste for them. Instead, put your efforts into having more broccoli, spinach, and winter squash, the richly colored, more nutrient-dense choices.

- Include lettuce, tomato, and green or red peppers on your sandwiches and wraps.
- Keep baby carrots, pepper strips, and cherry tomatoes handy in the front of the refrigerator for easy snacking. You'll be surprised how quickly they get eaten, particularly if you include hummus or a low-fat ranch dressing for a dip!
- Eat colorful salads filled with tomatoes, green peppers, carrots, spinach, and dark lettuces. Pale salads with white lettuce, cucumbers, onions, celery, and other pale veggies offer little more than crunch. When smothered with dressing, this crunch becomes highly caloric. At restaurants, alternatives to a pale salad include tomato juice, vegetable soup, a steamed veggie or, when you get home, a handful of raw baby carrots for a snack.
- Fortify spaghetti sauce with a box of frozen chopped broccoli, spinach, or green peppers. Cook the veggies alongside the spaghetti (in a steamer over the pasta water) or in the microwave before you add them to the tomato sauce.
- Choose fast foods with the most veggies:
  - pizza with peppers, mushrooms, and extra tomato sauce
  - Chinese entrées stir-fried with vegetables
  - lunchtime V-8 juice instead of diet soda
- Even over-cooked vegetables are better than no vegetables. If your only option is over-cooked veggies from the cafeteria, eat them. While cooking does destroy some of the vegetable's nutrients, it does not destroy all of them. Again, any vegetable is better than no vegetable.
- Keep frozen vegetables stocked in your freezer, ready and waiting. They are quick and easy to prepare, won't spoil quickly, and have more nutrients than "fresh" vegetables that have been in the store and your refrigerator for a few days.
- Because cooking reduces a vegetable's nutritional content:
  - Quickly steam vegetables only until tender crisp and instead of discarding cooking water, use it as a broth.
  - Microwave vegetables in a covered dish.
  - Stir-fry them with a little olive or canola oil.
- Use a blender or food processor to finely chop veggies to

include in meatloaf, soup, and stews. Or use packaged, pre-washed, and shredded cabbage, carrot, or broccoli, (found in your produce section) which are ready-to-go.

- When all else fails, eat fruit to help compensate for a lack of vegetables. The best alternatives include bananas, oranges, grapefruit, melon, strawberries, blueberries, and kiwi. These choices are rich in many of the same nutrients found in vegetables.

For more information on ways to add more fruits and vegetables to your daily diet, see: www.ChooseMyPlate.gov

● **PROTEIN FOR YOUR SPORTS DIET**—Like carbohydrates, protein-rich foods are an important part of your sports diet. You should eat a protein-rich food at each meal. Cyclists tend to either over- or under-consume protein. Some fill up on animal proteins like big burgers, slabs of steaks, eggs (or egg whites), and chicken, and get more than enough protein (and often,

way too much saturated fat). Others bypass these foods in their efforts to eat a low-fat, meat-free, or vegetarian diet, but neglect to eat adequate non-animal sources of protein, such as beans and tofu, resulting in a protein-deficient diet. For additional information and more specific guidelines on protein, see chapter 6.

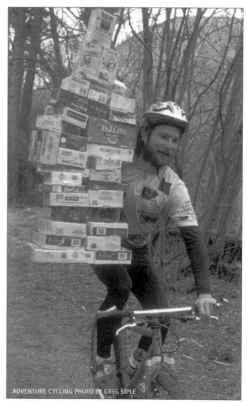

Protein comes from meat, fish, chicken, beans, tofu, and nuts, and also from calcium-rich milk, yogurt, cheese, and soy-alternatives. Getting enough calcium is necessary to maximize bone health and bone density, a particular concern for growing teens and women. Research shows that consuming calcium-rich foods may also play a role in facilitating weight loss and protecting against high blood pressure. Note that fat-

ADVENTURE CYCLING PHOTO BY GREG SIPLE

Balancing good nutrition and cycling does not have to be difficult. It just takes a little planning and practice.

The recommended daily calcium intake is:

Age Group	Calcium
Teens, 9-18 years	1,300 mg
Adults, 19-50 years	1,000 mg
Men 51-70 years	1,000 mg
Women, 51-70 years	1,200 mg
Adults, 71+ years	1,200 mg

Source: Institute of Medicine, 2010.

Each of the following foods provides about 300 milligrams of calcium. Three choices per day, or one at each meal, will contribute to meeting your calcium needs.

Calcium-rich Foods

Milk and milk products:	Amount
Milk	1 cup
Yogurt	1 cup
Cheese	1½ ounces
Cottage cheese	2 cups
Frozen yogurt	1½ cups

1 cup = 240 milliliters; 1 ounce = 28 grams or 30 milliliters. Nutrition information from USDA National Nutrient Database (online).

Proteins:	Amount
Soymilk	1 cup
Tofu	8 ounces (½ cake)
Salmon, canned with bones	5 ounces
Sardines, canned with bones	3 ounces
Almonds	4 ounces

Vegetables:	Amount
Broccoli, cooked	3 cups
Collard or turnip greens, cooked	1 cup
Kale or mustard greens, cooked	1½ cups

Many female athletes tend to consume a shockingly low amount of calcium. While we don't recommend supplements in place of food, if you won't consume a calcium-rich dairy food or a calcium fortified food (such as fortified orange juice or soymilk) with each meal, taking supplemental calcium, in combination with Vitamin D, is a smart idea.

free and low-fat products are preferable for heart health and calorie control, but you need not suffer with fat-free milk if you really don't like it. You can always cut back on fat in other foods in your diet. For example, have fat-free salad dressing or skip the butter on your dinner potato. For more information on dietary fat, see chapter 7.

Those who prefer a dairy-free diet or are lactose intolerant should take special care to eat adequate amounts of lactose-free or nondairy calcium sources. See *Calcium Equivalents* (above) for suggestions.

• **SWEETS AND TREATS**—Although nutritionists recommend eating a wholesome diet based on grains, fruits, and vegetables, some cyclists eat a diet with too many sweets and treats. If you have a junk-food diet, you may be able correct this imbalance by eating more wholesome foods *before you get too hungry*. Cyclists who get too hungry tend to choose sugary, fatty foods (such as apple pie, instead of apples). A simple solution to the junk-food diet is to *prevent* hunger by eating heartier portions of wholesome foods at meals.

Take note: You need not eat a "perfect diet" (*no* fats, *no* sugar) to have a good diet. Nothing is nutritionally wrong with having something sweet, such as a cookie for dessert after having eaten a sandwich, milk, and fruit for lunch. But a lot is wrong with eating cookies for lunch and skipping the sandwich. Ditto for living on gels and sports drinks for a day-long ride. That's when nutrition and performance problems arise.

The key to balancing fats and sugars appropriately in your diet is to abide by the following guidelines:

• Ten percent of your calories can appropriately come from refined sugar. That's about 200 to 300 calories from sugar per day for most cyclists. Take note: Gels and sports drinks count as refined sugar!

• Twenty-five percent of your calories can appropriately come from (preferably healthful) fat. That's about 450 to 750 calories from fat per day, or roughly 50–85 grams of fat per day.

Hence, moderate amounts of chips, cookies, and ice cream can fit into an overall healthful food plan, if desired. But be wise, and try to eat more of the best foods, and less of the rest.

Want some help shaping up your diet?

If you want personalized dietary advice, we recommend you seek professional advice from a registered dietitian (RD) who specializes in sports nutrition and, ideally, is Board Certified as a Specialist in Sports Dietetics (CSSD). To find a sports nutritionist in your area, use the referral networks at the American Dietetic Association's website (www.eatright.org) or the website of ADA's practice group of sports dietitians (www.SCANdpg.org). Or, try a web search by entering "sports nutritionist" and your city. You'll be glad you did! This personal nutrition coach can help you easily win with good nutrition.

● **SUMMARY**—Nutrition for cycling is all about eating with a purpose so you can then enjoy the benefits of high energy and good health. Your food goals are to eat:

- at least three kinds of wholesome foods at each meal
- at least two kinds of wholesome foods for each snack
- evenly-sized meals about every four hours throughout the day (as opposed to "crescendo eating" with a small breakfast and a large meal at the end of the day)
- and at least 85 to 90 percent of the calories from quality foods and, if desired, the remaining 10 to 15 percent from sweets and treats.

You need not eat a "perfect diet" to have a good diet, but you do want to choose more of the best foods (wholesome grains, fruits, vegetables, low-fat dairy products, and lean meats or beans) and less of the rest.

Words of wisdom from other cyclists... ━━━━━━━━━━━━━━━━

"I eat often, every two to three hours,
to keep my energy level up. Three meals alone would never do!"
MaryAnn Martinez, Concord, MA

"It's not just what I eat pre-ride and post-ride that impacts
my riding and performance; it's my overall everyday diet."
Maryann Martinez, Concord, MA

"We purchase a share in a local farm nearby through a local
CSA (community supported agriculture). We get a box of fresh fruits
and vegetables once per week and recipes in the newsletter.
As a result, we have learned to love all kinds of kale and other
vegetables that we otherwise would never have purchased."
Marcia Gibbs, California

"I try to live by the 90/10 rule: 90 percent of the time I eat nutritious food;
10 percent of the time I have fun foods as a reward for my hard training.
The 10 percent includes chocolate, beer, onion rings, blue cheese,
doughnuts, and ice cream."
Earl Fenstermacher, Seattle, WA

CHAPTER 2

Breakfast: The Meal of Champions

GOOD NUTRITION FOR CYCLISTS STARTS AT BREAKFAST. BREAKFAST IS the most important meal of your sports diet because it fuels your body and mind for a day of high energy and healthful eating. Yet many cyclists skip breakfast. They push themselves through their busy schedules and struggle with low energy, less-than-stellar riding, cravings for fatty sweets, hunger, and often unwanted weight gain. If you are a breakfast skipper, consider the following:

- Breakfast eaters consume a more healthful diet that has more fiber, calcium, iron, and whole grains and less fat than do breakfast skippers. As a result, they have a reduced risk of osteoporosis, heart disease, and anemia.
- Eating breakfast raises low morning blood sugar levels and improves wakefulness, mood, concentration, and productivity.
- Breakfast gives you a leg-up on fuel for your active day, tops off depleted glycogen stores, and gives you the energy and power to ride and work hard.
- Breakfast eaters are more successful with weight control.

● **EXCUSES, EXCUSES**—If breakfast is so good for us, then why do so many people skip it? There are plenty of excuses: no time, too busy, not hungry, you name it. But for every excuse to skip breakfast there is an even better reason not to.

Excuse: "I don't have time." If you have no time for breakfast, keep in mind that you can always make time to do what you want to do. A lack of priority may be the real problem, not

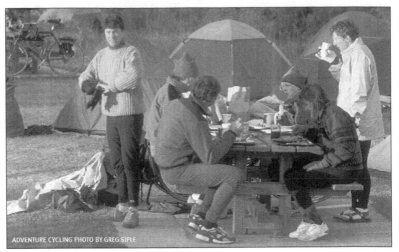

Enjoying a wholesome breakfast with friends is one of the pleasures of bike touring. For all cyclists, breakfast provides fuel for more energy and stronger riding.

a lack of time. Breakfast need not be elaborate. You can prepare and eat breakfast in mere minutes whether at home, at a campsite, or on the run:

- Get up ten minutes earlier to eat a bowl of cereal.
- Munch on a bagel and a banana as you break camp.
- Enjoy peanut butter on an English muffin as you get dressed.
- Sip on a smoothie or protein shake as you drive to work.

Here are a few quick, grab-and-go items for a healthy breakfast:

- Raisins or dried fruit and granola tossed into a plastic baggie
- Pita pocket with hummus or reduced-fat cheese
- A container of cottage cheese or yogurt
- Apple, orange, or banana plus a handful of crackers, nuts, or dry cereal
- Packets of instant oatmeal with an individual box of raisins
- Individual servings of juice, milk, or soymilk
- Toasted whole-grain waffles sandwiched with almond butter

The key to breakfast during the morning rush is to plan ahead. When touring, go food shopping the prior evening and stock up on breakfast staples. At home, prepare your breakfast the night before so you have it in a hurry: pour a bowl of cereal so all you have to do is add milk; set out the peanut butter jar and a sliced bagel; or pack a bag with yogurt and fruit and keep it in the refrigerator. Keep sliced bagels, bran muffins, and

Not everyone likes cereal for breakfast nor wants to cook eggs or pancakes. If what to eat for breakfast stumps you, choose a food that you enjoy. After all, you'll be more likely to eat breakfast if it tastes good. Remember that *any food*, even a cookie (preferably oatmeal raisin, rather than chocolate chip), is better than *no food*.

How about:
- Leftover pizza
- Leftover Chinese, Mexican, or other dinner food
- Mug of tomato soup
- Potato or sweet potato zapped in the microwave while you take your shower
- Tuna sandwich
- Peanut butter and apple
- Protein bar

sliced whole-grain breads in individual bags in the freezer; simply take one or two out of the freezer at night so breakfast is ready and waiting in the morning.

Excuse: "Breakfast interferes with my training schedule." If you are an early-morning rider, you will perform better and avoid an energy crash if you eat something beforehand. A quick meal of coffee with extra milk, a swig of juice, and a slice or two of toast contributes to greater stamina and helps you feel more awake. If you have trouble tolerating early-morning, pre-ride food, try consuming just a simple snack of easy-to-digest foods, such as an energy bar or some graham crackers. If you can tolerate no food, eat a hefty snack the night before, such as a sandwich, dinner leftovers, or a large bowl of cereal before bed.

Breakfast is equally important if you ride mid-day or in the afternoon. Eating breakfast tops off depleted glycogen stores and increases energy reserves to fuel mind and body during exercise. If you ride both in the morning and in the afternoon, eat breakfast before and after your morning ride (that is, enjoy two breakfasts). Because your muscles absorb the most carbohydrate within the first hour after hard exercise, a quick recovery breakfast is essential for a strong second workout.

Excuse: "I'm not hungry in the morning." If you have no morning appetite, the chances are you ate your breakfast calories the night before. Did you eat a huge dinner, lots of cookies, or a too many chips before bedtime? The solution to having no morning appetite is to eat less at night so you can start the day off hungry.

Some people find that training hard first thing in the morning kills their appetite. This lack of hunger is due to the rise in body temperature. Appetite should return within an hour after the body cools down. Plan ahead so that when hunger hits, healthful foods are ready and waiting. Otherwise, you are likely to grab whatever is easy, which may include doughnuts, pastries, and other high-fat foods with little nutritional value.

Excuse: "I'm on a diet." Too many weight-conscious cyclists start their diet at breakfast. Bad idea. People who skip breakfast tend to gain weight and be heavier than people who eat breakfast. Eating a satisfying breakfast prevents you from becoming overly hungry and overeating. Breakfast gives you the energy to ride harder and longer so you burn more calories and improve your physical condition.

Many breakfast skippers believe they will eat more calories and gain weight if they eat breakfast. Consider this: Dieters who skip breakfast tend to eat the majority of their day's calories in the evening. They eat dinner then have the "munchies" all evening. They end up snacking on large amounts of sweets, ice cream, or chips until bedtime. They wake up with a food hangover, skip breakfast, and perpetuate the cycle.

If this sounds familiar, you would be better off shifting some of those evening calories to a bigger breakfast and lunch. You'll have more energy when you need it most: during the day and during your ride. You'll be less hungry in the evening so you can then eat a sensible dinner and avoid the post-dinner munchies that can ruin a sports diet. Chapter 16 has more details about how to lose weight and have energy to train.

Excuse: "Breakfast makes me hungrier." Some cyclists complain that if they eat breakfast, they become hungrier than if they skipped breakfast and they believe they end up eating more all day. This may result from thinking they have already "blown" their diets by eating breakfast, so they might as well keep overeating and then start dieting again the next day. Wrong. If you feel hungry after breakfast, you probably ate too little. One hundred calories of toast with jam merely whets your appetite and does not satisfy your calorie needs.

Try budgeting about one-quarter of your day's calories for breakfast: about 500 to 600 calories for most 120- to 150-pound cyclists. This translates into two slices of toast, two poached eggs, a banana, and a low-fat latte; or yogurt and a bagel with peanut butter. If that is too much food for you to eat in one sitting, split it in half and enjoy two smaller breakfasts: Eat a first breakfast a 7 a.m. and a second breakfast at 9:30 a.m. Be sure to include some protein-rich food in your breakfast. It's satisfying and will keep you feeling "fed."

It is far better to consume your calories during the day when your body needs them than to wait until evening when you are winding down for the night. If you eat enough at breakfast you will not be as hungry for dinner and will be able to eat smaller portions. See chapter 15 for more information on how to calculate your calorie needs.

● **THE BREAKFAST OF CHAMPIONS**—By now we hope we have convinced you that breakfast is indeed the most important meal of the day. What is best to eat, you wonder? As a general rule, you should choose at least three different kinds of foods (such as grain + milk + fruit). We highly recommend a wholesome cereal as the breakfast of champions for several reasons. Cereal is:

- *Nutritious.* A bowl of whole-grain cereal with fruit and low-fat milk supplies calcium, fiber, and other nutrients active people need. Iron-fortified cereals provide a source of iron to help reduce your risk of becoming anemic.
- *Carbohydrate-rich.* Your brain and muscles need carbohydrates to work well. A bowl of cereal with milk and banana supplies you with three good sources of carbohydrates.
- *Quick, easy, and portable.* With cereal in your kitchen cupboard, desk drawer, pannier, or travel bag, you will always have a no-mess, no-cook, high-carbohydrate meal or snack to eat.
- *Versatile.* You can eat it dry if you're on the run or preferably with low-fat milk or yogurt to add protein and calcium. It

Needless to say, all cereals are not created equal. By reading the Nutrition Facts on the cereal box, you can see that some offer more nutritional value than others. Here are four tips to help you make the best cereal choices:

1. *Choose iron-enriched cereals with at least 25 percent of the Daily Value for iron to help prevent anemia.*

    Note, however, the iron in breakfast cereals is poorly absorbed compared to the iron in lean red meats. But you can enhance iron absorption by drinking a glass of orange juice or enjoying another source of vitamin C (such as grapefruit, cantaloupe, strawberries, or kiwi) along with the cereal. And *any* iron is better than no iron.

    If you tend to eat "all-natural" types of cereals, such as granola and shredded wheat, be aware that these types have "no additives," hence no added iron. You might want to mix and match all-natural brands with iron-enriched brands (or make the effort to eat iron-rich foods at other meals).

2. *Choose fiber-rich cereals with more than 5 grams of fiber per serving.*

    Fiber not only helps prevent constipation but is also a protective nutrient that may reduce your risk of colon cancer and heart disease. Whole-grain and bran cereals are the best sources of fiber, more so than even fruits and vegetables. Choose from All-Bran, Raisin Bran, Bran Chex, Fiber One, or any of the numerous cereals with "bran" or "fiber" in the name. You can also mix together high- and low-fiber cereals (for example, Rice Krispies + Fiber One; Special K + Raisin

also makes a good snack. You can mix brands and vary the flavor with different toppings:
–Yogurt or vanilla soymilk
–Chopped dates or dried apricots
–Dried cranberries and sunflower seeds
–Brown sugar or maple syrup
–Sliced fresh apple or peach
–Walnuts, cinnamon, and sliced banana
–Peanut or almond butter and cinnamon (for hot cereal)
–Applesauce and brown sugar (for hot cereal)
–Pumpkin (canned), cinnamon, and brown sugar (for hot cereal)
–Frozen berries: Nancy's favorite is to put a mix of cereals in a bowl, top it with frozen blueberries, heat it in the microwave oven for 30 to 60 seconds, and then add cold milk. It is like eating fruit cobbler!

Bran). Fiber-rich cereal is good for cyclists because it offers sustained energy, more so than refined grains, and thus fuels you for the long run. Note: If you have trouble with diarrhea when cycling, you may want to forgo bran cereals! The extra fiber may aggravate the situation.

3. *Choose cereals with whole grains listed among the first ingredients.*

Whole grains include whole wheat, brown rice, corn, and oats; these should be listed first in the ingredients. Pay more attention to a cereal's grain content than its sugar or sodium (salt) content. Sugar is a simple carbohydrate that fuels your muscles. Yes, sugar calories are nutritionally empty calories. But when they are combined with milk, banana, and the cereal itself, the twenty empty calories in five grams of added sugar are insignificant. Obviously, sugar-filled frosted flakes and kids' cereals with 15 grams of sugar or more per serving are more like dessert than breakfast. Hence, try to limit your breakfast choices to cereals with fewer than 5 grams of added sugar per serving. Enjoy the sugary ones for snacks or dessert, if desired, or mix a little with low-sugar cereals.

4. *Choose primarily low-fat cereals with less than 2 grams of fat per serving.*

High-fat cereals such as some brands of granola and crunchy cookie-type cereals can add unexpected fat and calories to your sports diet. Select low-fat brands for the foundation of your breakfast and then use only a sprinkling of the higher-fat treats, if desired, for a topping.

Other good breakfast choices include wholesome carbohydrate-rich foods, such as whole-grain bagels, pancakes, whole-wheat toast, fresh fruit, low-fat yogurt and milk, and low-fat bran muffins. Greasy bacon-and-egg meals or low-carb, egg white-and-veggie omelets lack the carbohydrates you need to optimally fuel your muscles with glycogen. Of course, eating anything, even a bowl of frozen yogurt or a couple of cookies, is better than eating nothing.

● **BREAKFAST ON THE ROAD**—At a restaurant, you can be confronted with fat-laden cheese omelets, hash browns, sausage, and buttery toast. Take the higher-carbohydrate route by ordering a fruit cup, oatmeal, and/or poached eggs and whole-wheat bagel with jam. If you want a bigger breakfast, enjoy pancakes (increasingly available in whole-wheat) or French toast. Order a

● MIX 'N MATCH CEREALS

When it comes to cereals, you may not find the ideal cereal that meets all of your standards for high fiber, high iron, and low fat, but you can always mix-and-match to create a winning combination. The list below highlights how different cereals offer different benefits. Check the nutritional labels of your favorites as well.

Brand	Iron (%DV*)	Fiber (g)	Fat (g)
The "ideal cereal"	›25%	›5	‹2.0
Cheerios, 1 cup (30 g)	45%	3	2.0
Wheaties, 1 cup (30 g)	45%	3	1.0
Kashi Go Lean, 1 cup (50 g)	10%	10	1.0
Kellogg's Raisin Bran, 1 cup (60 g)	25%	7	1.5
Fiber One, ½ cup (30 g)	25%	14	1.0
Quaker 100% Natural, ½ cup (50 g)	6%	3	6.0
Quaker Oat Squares, 1 cup (60 g)	80%	4	2.5

*%DV (percent Daily Value) is a guide to the nutrients found in one serving of food. For example, if the food label lists 45% DV for iron, you'll get 45% of the iron you need for the day. (The DV for iron is 18 milligrams.) A food is considered to be low in a nutrient if it offers 5% or less of that nutrient. It's considered to be high if it offers 20% or more.

Nutrition information from food labels.

large orange juice or tomato juice, to help compensate for a potential lack of fruits or veggies in the other meals.

What about coffee?—Some cyclists hop out of bed ready to jump into a busy day. Others search for a morning cup of coffee or other caffeinated beverage to help start their engines. Caffeine is a proven energy enhancer, which is further discussed in chapter 9.

Little is wrong with enjoying some morning brew especially if you use milk instead of cream or creamer; a lot is wrong if you rely on caffeine instead of food for energy. Be sure to enjoy at least a granola bar along with the coffee. Also make the effort to get adequate sleep so you have less need for a caffeine wake-up. The same holds true of tea. For a more nourishing hot beverage, enjoy some hot chocolate made with milk or soymilk.

Have you developed a "Starbuck's habit"? If so, take note: The specialty coffee drinks contain not only caffeine but often enough calories from cream and sugar to equal a small to medium meal, and an unhealthful one at that. Understand what you are ordering, and make it a good choice, such as a decaf skim milk latte or skim milk hot chocolate.

● SUMMARY—

- What you eat in the morning provides fuel for a high-energy day.
- The best choices for breakfast include wholesome carbohydrate-based foods such as cereal with milk, fruit, and whole-grain bagels. But remember, eating or drinking anything is better than consuming nothing.
- Food in the morning provides fuel for more energy and stronger workouts, essential for improving your fitness level and cycling performance.
- Dieters can enjoy breakfast without the fear of sabotaging their diets. Breakfast curbs evening appetite so dieters can eat lighter at night and lose weight when they are sleeping, not biking.
- If you generally skip breakfast, at least give breakfast a try on the days you ride. You'll soon learn why breakfast is the meal of champions! See chapter 10 for more on the importance of pre-ride food.

Words of wisdom from other cyclists... ━━━━━━━━━

"My favorite breakfast is hot oatmeal with a spoonful of canned pumpkin or frozen berries, and a dash of cinnamon and brown sugar. It tastes great and I get a jump on my fruit and vegetable intake before 8 a.m."
Paul Humphries, Reading, MA

"When my legs feel like mud, I know I didn't eat enough breakfast."
Rich Lesnik, San Francisco, CA

"For training rides that will go longer than 4 hours, I set the alarm for 4 a.m. I get up to eat a hearty breakfast, and then I go back to sleep until I have to get up. This ensures I'm topped off before the big ride."
Khai Harbut, Plano, TX

CHAPTER 3

Lunch, Snacks, and Dinner

GIVEN THAT LUNCH, SNACKS, AND DINNER SUPPLY THE MAJORITY OF your day's calories, you should wisely choose these foods to assure you are consuming an optimal sports diet. A good rule of thumb is to choose at least three (preferably four) different kinds of foods for a meal and at least two kinds of foods for a snack:

- *Lunch:* whole-grain bread + turkey + low-fat cheese + apple
- *Snack:* graham crackers + peanut butter
- *Dinner:* spaghetti + tomato sauce + meatballs + low-fat milk

Because good nutrition starts in the supermarket, you have a far better chance of achieving a super sports diet when your kitchen is well-stocked with appropriate foods. You might want to make a copy of the Cyclist's Basic Shopping List (page 32) and post it on your refrigerator.

Meal Timing—You should plan to eat at least every four hours throughout the day based on your hunger and physical desire to eat. While bike touring, you'll want to eat at least every two hours. Don't ignore your hunger and go too long between meals. That is, if you are hungry by 10 a.m., do not wait until "lunchtime" to eat at noon. That's counter to your goals of enjoying a high-energy day.

Hunger is simply your body's request for more fuel. Denying food can lead to lags in energy, sweet cravings, extreme hunger and then overeating. As an active cyclist, you can expect to get hungry at least every two to four hours, and you should plan your meals accordingly. If you eat a pre-ride breakfast at 7 a.m., you can appropriately be hungry for a second breakfast at 9 a.m., and then a lunch at noon—with a snack in between if you are on a long ride.

Plan to distribute your day's calories evenly among your meals. Each meal or section of the day—morning, noon, and evening—should provide you with approximately the same number of calories. Lots of cyclists and other active people eat too little at breakfast and lunch, only to consume most of their day's calorie budget after 5 p.m. But why wait until evening to eat when you could have used those calories to energize your day and your workout?

If you generally wait until the end of your day to enjoy a big meal, you may want to rethink your eating plan. Here are two sample eating templates for a cyclist who needs 2,400 calories a day (such as a 120-pound woman who rides for 60 to 90 minutes):

Four Meals a Day			Five Meals a Day		
Meal	Time	Calories	Meal	Time	Calories
Breakfast	7 a.m.	600	Breakfast	7 a.m.	600
First lunch	10 a.m.	600	Snack	10 a.m.	300
Second lunch	2 p.m.	600	Lunch	1 p.m.	600
Dinner	6 p.m.	600	Snack	4 p.m.	300
			Dinner	7 p.m.	600

• **LUNCH**—Whereas breakfast is the most important meal of the day, lunch is the second most important. Breakfast fills your tank with fuel; lunch replenishes it. Lunch renews glycogen stores drained by morning activities and provides fuel for the afternoon. Cyclists who skip or skimp on lunch compromise their training and their enjoyment of a day-long tour by:
• not being properly fueled for the afternoon or evening ride,
• getting overly hungry and gorging on goodies all evening, and
• missing out on the nutrients muscles need to recover from a morning workout.

Brown-Bagging It—If you are organized enough to make your own lunch, bringing it with you is the best option for many reasons. It saves money (you don't have to order out), saves time (you don't have to head to the cafeteria), and can be more nutritious compared to high-fat restaurant food. The key is to make lunch preparation fast and simple. See *Brown-Bag Lunches* on page 25 for helpful tips.

Fast-Food Meals—Unfortunately, few cyclists make the effort to organize their lunch plans in advance of noontime. If that describes you, fast food can save the day—or it can spoil your sports diet. The traditional fast-food meal is loaded with fat, sodium, and cholesterol and is low in fiber. The good news is that most quick-service restaurants now offer healthful options: low-fat chicken sandwiches, hearty soups, salads, and even vegetarian burgers. Though you may be tempted to order a deluxe burger and fries, remind yourself that you will be healthier, feel better, and feel better about yourself if you forgo the grease and order the healthful option. Below are suggestions for lower-fat meals found at popular quick-service restaurants. Chapter 14 offers more information about restaurant eating.

Dunkin' Donuts:	Low-fat muffin, bagel, juice, bean or broth-based soups, hot cocoa, bagel-and-egg sandwich
Deli:	Bagel with bean- or broth-based soups; sandwiches or subs with lots of bread and half the roast beef, turkey, ham, or cheese. Or, ask for two extra slices of bread or a second roll to make a sandwich for your second lunch with the excessive meat. Go light on the mayonnaise, and instead, add moistness with sliced tomatoes, lettuce, mustard, or ketchup. Add more carbohydrates with juice, fruit, fig bars, or yogurt for dessert.
McDonald's:	Sandwich with grilled chicken, yogurt parfait, salad with dressing on the side
Wendy's:	Bowl of chili with a plain baked potato
Taco Bell:	Bean burrito or soft chicken taco with extra lettuce and tomato. Limit cheese and sour cream.
Pizza:	Thick-crust with extra veggies or a side salad rather than extra cheese or pepperoni or other fatty meat

The following suggestions may help you pack a super sports lunch.

- Make lunch the night before to reduce chaos in your morning rush hour.

- To keep sandwich bread fresh, store it in the freezer and take out the slices as needed. Bread thaws in minutes at room temperature or in seconds in the microwave oven.

- Make several sandwiches at once and store them in the freezer. Grab one on your way out the door. The frozen sandwich will be thawed and fresh by lunchtime. Sliced meats and peanut butter freeze nicely. Don't freeze eggs, mayonnaise, or raw vegetables.

- Try different low-fat sandwich spreads: low-fat or fat-free mayonnaise, plain yogurt or yogurt/mayonnaise mixtures, low-fat or fat-free salad dressings, honey-mustard, salsa, or hummus.

- Add a good helping of lettuce and tomato to a sandwich for a full serving of vegetables.

- Buy pre-washed fresh vegetables, such as peeled baby carrots, salad, broccoli florets, shredded cabbage, coleslaw mix, and carrots to save time and hassle. Toss a variety together for a quick salad or add them to sandwiches, roll-ups, or pita pockets.

- Liven up an old-fashioned peanut butter sandwich by adding sliced banana or apple, raisins, or dates.

- Slice low-fat cheese, store it in a sealed container or plastic bag, and keep it in the refrigerator. Make a meat-free sandwich with cheese, peppers, avocado, and sprouts.

- Keep a tub of hummus in the refrigerator and a package of (preferably whole-wheat) lavash, pita bread, or flour tortillas in the freezer. Thaw the bread or tortilla in the microwave, add hummus and a combination of pre-washed raw vegetables, and roll it up for a tasty vegetarian wrap.

- Keep a bowl of fresh fruit, like bananas, oranges, and washed apples, pears, and plums, on the kitchen counter or in your desk at work for easy access.

- Stock up on individual containers of yogurt, cottage cheese, canned fruit, pudding, 100% fruit and vegetable juices, and string cheese to toss in your lunch bag.

- At dinner, cook extra so you have leftovers for tomorrow's lunch. Distribute the food among a few small microwaveable containers, making several complete meals, and store them in the refrigerator or freezer. This way, a balanced meal of soup, chili, pasta, or meat and potatoes is on hand for you to grab and go.

Pasta:	Spaghetti or ziti with tomato sauce and grilled chicken or meatballs
Chinese:	Hot and sour or wonton soup; plain rice with stir-fried entrées such as beef and broccoli, or chicken with pea pods. Request the food be cooked with minimal oil. Limit fried appetizers and fried entrées and fill up on steamed rice (preferably brown rice) instead.
Soups:	Hearty soups (such as split pea, minestrone, lentil, vegetable, or noodle) accompanied by whole-grain crackers, roll, bagel, or English muffins
Beverages:	Milk—regular or soy, plain or flavored, preferably low-fat—is nutrient dense and a smart addition to a sports diet. Juices and sugar-filled soft drinks are both rich in carbohydrates that fuel muscles. Juices, however, are better for your health; 100% juice offers vitamin C and potassium, and provides wholesome goodness. Choose 100% natural juices instead of "vitamin waters."

Salad for Lunch—Salads, whether served as a main dish or an accompaniment, are a simple way to boost your intake of fresh vegetables—that's good! But most salads get the bulk of their calories from salad oil—not good. As an athlete, you need a substantial, carbohydrate-based lunch. You will fuel your muscles better if you choose a sandwich with a side salad for lunch rather than just a big salad for the entire meal. However, if salad is your choice, turn it into a substantial meal by topping your salad with foods rich in carbohydrates and protein (see number 2 below).

Three tricks to making a healthy sport salad are:
1. *Choose a variety of colorful vegetables*—dark green lettuces, red tomatoes, yellow peppers, and orange carrots—for a variety of vitamins and minerals. If the vegetables you buy for salads tend to wilt in your refrigerator, consider frequent trips to the salad bar at the grocery store and deli as an alternative

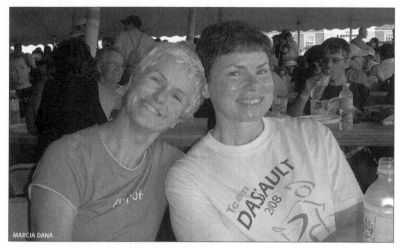

Eating wholesome meals both on the road and during events will contribute to radiant health as well as happy memories.

to tossing veggies that spoil before you find the chance to eat them. And here's a tip: Dig from the bottom to make sure to get the coldest (and therefore best preserved) part of the salad bar.

2. ***Add extra carbohydrates and some protein:***
   - Dense vegetables, such as corn, peas, beets, carrots
   - Beans and legumes, such as chickpeas, kidney beans, and three-bean salad
   - Cooked rice or pasta
   - Oranges, apples, grapes, raisins, or dried cranberries
   - Toasted croutons
   - Whole-grain bread or roll on the side
   - Hard-boiled eggs, cheese (moderate amounts), chicken, flaked tuna or imitation seafood, preferably without mayonnaise

3. ***Monitor the dressing.*** Some cyclists drown 50 calories of healthful salad ingredients with 400 calories of blue cheese dressing! At a restaurant always request the dressing be served on the side. Otherwise, you may get 400 calories of oil or mayonnaise, fatty foods that fill your stomach but leave your muscles unfueled.

   If you choose regular dressings, select those made with olive or canola oil for flavor and for their health-protective

● SALADS

Here are how some popular salad ingredients compare. Those with the most color generally have the most nutritional value.

Salad Ingredient	Vitamin C (mg)	Vitamin A (IU)	Magnesium (mg)
Daily Value (recommended intake)	60	5,000	400
Broccoli, 5-inch (13 cm) stalk (180 g)	110	2,500	24
Green pepper, ½ (70 g)	65	210	20
Spinach, 2 cups raw (110 g)	50	8,100	90
Tomato, medium (12 g)	25	760	15
Romaine, 2 cups (110 g)	30	3,000	10
Iceberg, 2 cups (110 g)	5	360	5
Cucumber, ½ medium (150 g)	10	325	15
Celery, 1 stalk (40 g)	5	55	4

Nutrition information from USDA National Nutrient Database (online).

mono- and poly-unsaturated fats. If you want to reduce your fat intake, you can dilute regular dressings with water, vinegar, lemon, or milk. (Milk works best for ranch and creamy-style dressings.) Or, you can choose from the plethora of reduced-fat or fat-free salad dressings. These are good not only for salads but also sandwiches, baked potatoes, and dips.

● SNACKS—In many countries such as England or Germany, an afternoon cup of tea or coffee along with a sweet is tradition-al. This scheduled snack provides a pleasant break as well as an energy booster. In comparison, many Americans believe snacking between meals is sinful; if they succumb to eating, they feel guilty.

One reason people think snacking is bad is because they snack on candy, cookies, doughnuts, or chips. These foods pro-vide few nutrients needed for optimal cycling performance. A better choice is to trade 250 calories of a candy bar for 250 calo-ries of nuts and raisins. Appropriate snacking refuels you, gives you necessary nutrients, and gives you extra energy to perform your best on the bike. Snacking can be good for you and should be a part of your training and touring diet.

Or instead of snacking, why not think about eating two lunches! For instance, have a first lunch at 11:00 a.m. when you first start to get hungry and then a second lunch at 3:00 p.m.. That way you can enjoy a meal when the afternoon munchies strike and there's time for it to digest before you ride at 4:30 or 5:00 p.m. This two-lunch plan helps you refuel from a morning ride and prepares you for a strong late-afternoon ride. If you ride in early afternoon, like at 3:00 p.m., you may want to divide your second lunch into smaller pre- and post-exercise snacks. In all cases, two lunches will curb your appetite so you are not starving at the end of the day.

Experiment with this two-lunch concept. If you are like most hungry cyclists, you'll find yourself looking forward to a second sandwich to boost your energy. Plus, it prevents the hungry horrors that can sidetrack all your good intentions at dinnertime.

Afraid that two lunches will be too much food? Fear not; a second lunch does not mean additional calories. You'll simply be trading your afternoon cookies and evening ice cream for a wholesome afternoon meal. You'll curb your cravings for evening snacks—you ate them earlier in the day (in the form of wholesome foods).

What to Eat for Your Second Lunch—A second lunch does not have to be a hassle. The easier it is, the more likely you are to eat it. You want something you can consume in a matter of a few minutes; it really doesn't take long to enjoy a peanut butter sandwich and a yogurt at your desk. The key is to plan ahead to have foods available.

- Keep foods that are not highly perishable in your car, desk drawer, backpack, gym bag, or handlebar bag: dried fruit, nuts, energy bars, granola bars, crackers, pretzels, fig bars, oatmeal-raisin cookies, graham crackers, trail mix, V-8 juice, and juice boxes.
- If you pack a lunch bag, include a second sandwich.
- Use the office refrigerator to store a stash of yogurt, cottage cheese, juice, cheese sticks, and baby carrots.
- Consider a liquid meal such as a fruit smoothie, protein shake, or instant breakfast drink.

Some cyclists enjoy a second sandwich for their second lunch. But others prefer two or three of the wholesome snacks listed here. Keep healthful snacks on hand at work, in your bike bag, or in your car so you can avoid the temptations that lurk in every corner store, vending machine, or bakery. For the most nutrition, pick two or three different foods for each snack, such as carrots + cottage cheese + crackers; or graham crackers + peanut butter + apple.

Perishable snacks to keep in the refrigerator at work, portable cooler, or thermal lunch bag:

- Whole-wheat bagel
- Low-fat bran muffin
- Microwaved potato or sweet potato
- Low-fat yogurt, regular or Greek-style
- Low-fat cottage cheese
- Low-fat cheese sticks
- Thick-crust pizza
- Fresh fruit
- Baby carrots
- Leftover pasta
- Frozen meal
- Hard boiled egg
- Low-fat or fat-free milk and chocolate milk

Nonperishable snacks to keep in your desk drawer, backpack, or bike bag:

- Cold cereal
- Hot cereal
- Reduced-fat microwave popcorn
- Canned soup
- Canned tuna
- Low-fat whole-grain crackers
- Graham crackers
- Low-fat granola bars
- Energy bars
- Juice boxes or bottles
- Dried fruit
- Peanut butter
- Nuts, trail mix

Vending-Machine Options—By having a second lunch, you can reduce trips to the vending machines. But if you haven't prepared a second lunch and are faced with "machine cuisine," choose carefully! Tucked among the lackluster options, you may be able to find healthy options like pretzels, peanuts, juice, yogurt, or even an apple. The good part about vending-machine snacks is their limited size: A package of cookies contains three cookies rather than two dozen and generally provides only 200 to 400 calories, not 2,000.

If you're trying to decide between fatty or sugary choices (such as chips vs. jellybeans), remember that the sugar in jellybeans appropriately fuels your muscles, whereas the fat in the chips fills your stomach but leaves your muscles unfueled. To protect your teeth, be sure to brush or rinse your teeth after eating a sugary snack.

Treats—If it's an ice cream sundae or other such belt-busting treat that you are craving, why not satisfy your hankering by indulging at lunchtime rather than at dinnertime or later? By spending your lunchtime calories on the treat, you can still balance the rest of your day's calorie and nutrition budget—and you'll certainly have incentive to train harder that afternoon! You won't destroy your health with an occasional treat as long as your overall diet tends to be wholesome.

• **DINNER**—Dinnertime generally marks the end of the day's work, a time to relax and enjoy a nice meal—that is, if you have the energy to prepare it. The challenge is to arrive at home or at the campground not starving and with enough energy to prepare a decent, healthy meal. This means eating at least 75 percent of your calories during the day as breakfast, lunch #1, and lunch #2.

If you are far from being a master chef, you might want to take a cooking class at your local center for adult education. You can also find basic cooking classes and easy recipes on the Internet. Touring cyclists might want to pick up a camping cookbook prior to the tour. But remember, no number of cooking classes or recipes will help if you enter the dinner hour too hungry to cook or make wise food choices. And you won't be able to cook anything if you have failed to food shop, so be sure to plan "food shopping" into your schedule. Good nutrition starts in the grocery store!

Quick Fixes for Dinner—To make dinner preparation as hassle-free as possible when at home, you may want to incorporate some of the evening prep work into your morning routine. For example, while you shower or shave for work, you could cook a pot of rice or bake a potato. On days you don't want to cook, grocery stores offer convenient ready-to-eat meals, such as hot entrées and side dishes, soup-and-salad bars, deli sandwiches, and rotisserie chicken. These also offer a convenient option for touring cyclists who occasionally may not feel like getting out the camp stove.

Cupboard:
- hot and cold cereal
- spaghetti (whole-wheat or regular)
- egg noodles
- spaghetti sauce
- brown rice
- crackers
- kidney beans
- baked beans
- refried beans
- peanut butter
- soups (mushroom for making casseroles, lentil, minestrone, hearty bean)
- V-8 or other 100% vegetable juices
- raisins
- dried apricots or apples, nonperishable snack foods (see page 30 *Some Super Sport Snacks*)
- canned salmon
- sardines
- tuna
- olive oil and canola oil
- your favorite seasonings (garlic, cinnamon, soy sauce, etc.)
- nuts

Countertop:
- bananas
- tomatoes
- oranges
- russet and sweet potatoes (for baking)
- onions

Refrigerator:
- reduced-fat cheese
- low-fat cottage cheese
- low-fat milk
- soymilk
- low-fat yogurt
- Parmesan cheese
- eggs
- tofu
- tempeh
- flour and corn tortillas
- salad fixings
- carrots
- Romaine lettuce
- apples
- grapes
- hummus
- salsa
- 100% fruit juices
- sliced deli turkey and lean roast beef
- reduced-fat salad dressing
- reduced-fat mayonnaise
- your favorite condiments (mustard, jellies, ketchup, etc.)

Freezer:
- whole-grain bagels
- whole-wheat pita
- English muffins
- multigrain bread and hamburger buns
- low-fat bran muffins
- orange juice concentrate
- broccoli
- spinach
- winter squash
- peas

- corn
- blueberries or other fruit
- ground turkey
- extra-lean hamburger
- chicken (pieces frozen individually)
- seafood
- veggie or soy burgers

Menu Ideas:
If you keep these food stocked in your kitchen, you will have the makings for at least a week of simple, carbohydrate-based meals:
- pasta with tomato and meat, seafood, or beans
- quick stir-fry
- easy casseroles like tuna or chicken noodle
- homemade pizzas
- a variety of soups and hot or cold sandwiches
- meat or vegetarian burritos or tacos
- baked potatoes with your choice of hearty toppings
- meal-sized salads with veggies, pasta, and protein
- hearty hot or cold sandwiches

Here are some ideas for quick and easy meals:
- Pasta with clam sauce, tomato sauce, and/or frozen vegetables, and/or reduced-fat cheese
- Canned beans, rinsed and then spooned over rice, pasta, or salads
- Frozen dinners supplemented with whole-grain bread and fresh fruit
- Pierogies, tortellini, and burritos from the frozen food section, plus a side salad from the deli
- Baked potato topped with cottage cheese or ricotta
- Whole-grain cereal (hot or cold) with fruit and low-fat milk
- Quick-cooking brown rice. Make double for the next day's rice-and-bean salad.
- Stir-fry veggies and meat: Use precut vegetables from the market, salad bar, or freezer, leftover rice, and leftover meats. Use soy sauce, bottled stir-fry sauce from the supermarket, or garlic sauce purchased at any take-out Chinese restaurant.
- Scrambled eggs: Combine beaten eggs and seasonings with grated raw zucchini, reduced-fat cheese, tomato slices, or leftover cooked vegetables.
- Thick-crust pizza, fresh or frozen, reheated in the toaster oven
- Homemade pizza: pizza dough from the supermarket + jarred spaghetti sauce + steamed or sliced fresh veggies + grated low-fat cheese
- Bean soups: homemade, canned, or from the deli
- Souped-up soup: canned soup + added steamed vegetables, leftover meat or fish, or reduced-fat cheese

Rice and Cyclists—Rice is underrated as a sports food. Overshadowed by the more popular dinner starches (like potato and pasta), rice is a rich source of carbohydrates. Preferably you will choose brown rice instead of the refined, white varieties. When you cook rice, make extra. This way, cooked rice is on hand for quick dinner preparation. Come dinnertime, you can simply brown one pound of lean hamburger or ground turkey in a large skillet, dump in the cooked rice, and then add whatever vegetable is handy. Cooking 1½ cups of raw rice for each pound of raw lean meat generates two generous sports meals (or four average-sized meals) with 60 percent of the calories from carbohydrates. Perfect!

Some popular creations with rice and ground meat include:

- *Mexican*—canned beans + chili powder + grated low-fat cheese + diced tomatoes
- *Chinese*—broccoli zapped in the microwave oven while the meat cooks + soy sauce
- *Italian*—green beans + Italian seasonings such as basil, oregano, and garlic powder
- *American*—grated low-fat Cheddar cheese + onion browned with the meat + diced or canned tomatoes

Pasta and Cyclists—Every biker, regardless of language, understands the word pasta. Pasta parties are universally enjoyed around the world, and many cyclists consider pasta as the preferred food for carbo-loading and recovery. Indeed, many believe pasta to be some kind of super food, which it is not. Granted, pasta and most other noodles, such as rice, egg, or Chinese noodles, are carbohydrate-rich, easy to cook, economical, and enjoyed by almost every family member. But in terms of vitamins, minerals, fiber, and protein, plain pasta and noodles are lackluster foods.

Nutritional Value—Pasta is made from refined or processed flour, wheat that has been stripped of its fiber-rich bran and nutrient-rich germ. With respect to nutrition, plain pasta is really no different than soft white sandwich bread. Whole-wheat pasta, on the other hand, offers more nutrition, most notably fiber. If you don't like the taste or consistency of whole-wheat pasta, try mixing it with some traditional pasta.

Don't bank on spinach, tomato, or other such colorful pasta noodles to provide you with much added nutrition. These contain relatively little actual spinach or tomato, probably a teaspoon or less per cup of cooked pasta, and do not compare nutritionally to a one-cup serving of vegetables eaten with the meal.

The nutritional quality of your pasta meal can go up or down depending on what you add to your pasta. Pasta can be a fat-laden nutritional nightmare if it is smothered with butter, oil, cream sauce, or greasy meat sauces. Or it can be a nutritional super food if topped with vegetable sauces or lean meat or fish sauces:

Topping	Nutrients
• Tomato sauce, canned or homemade	Vitamins A and C, Potassium
• Pesto sauce made from fresh basil or spinach	Vitamins A and C, Potassium
• Sautéed bell peppers, tomato, and onion	Vitamins A and C, Potassium
• Tomato sauce with chicken, lean ground beef or turkey, clams, shrimp, or fish	Protein, Zinc, Iron, Vitamins A and C, Potassium
• Clam sauce made with a little olive oil	Protein, Zinc, Iron

Pasta and Protein—Pasta is popular not only for carbohydrates but also for being a vegetarian alternative to meat-based meals. However, many cyclists and other athletes live on too much pasta and neglect their protein needs. For example, Joe, an aspiring Olympian, thought his high-carbohydrate, low-fat diet of pasta and tomato sauce seven nights per week was top-notch. He wondered why he felt chronically tired and was not improving despite hard training. The answer was simple. His limited diet was deficient in protein, iron, and zinc. He resolved the problem by adding a variety of protein-rich choices to his tomato sauce:
- 2 to 3 ounces cooked extra-lean ground beef or turkey
- ¼ cup grated part-skim mozzarella cheese
- ½ cake tofu or tempeh
- ²/₃ cup canned, drained kidney or garbanzo beans
- 3 ounces tuna (half of a 6-ounce can)
- ½ cup canned clams or shrimp
- 1 cup low-fat cottage cheese

Or instead of adding protein to the sauce, he would drink two glasses of low-fat milk with the meal. Once he started to supplement the pasta with a variety of proteins, he started to feel better, train and perform better, and recover better.

Spuds for Cyclists—Potatoes are a good sports food for meals and snacks. Some cyclists carry baked potatoes in a pocket, as they might a piece of fruit, and munch on them during and after workouts when they need an energy boost.

Potatoes are rich in carbohydrates, potassium, and vitamin C. A large baked potato offers 65 percent the recommended daily intake for vitamin C and all the potassium you'd lose in three hours of sweaty exercise. A sweet potato offers the additional health benefits of beta-carotene. A large restaurant-size baked potato generally has around 200 calories. A restaurant's mashed potato, however, can contain upwards of 300 calories per cup because of the added butter and/or cream.

Here are some tips for enjoying both white and sweet potatoes:
- Russets are better suited for baking than red, white, or gold potatoes, which are preferred for boiling or mashing.
- Store potatoes at room temperature. Refrigerated potatoes quickly become sweet and off-colored.
- Eat the skin (even on sweet potatoes). You'll get more vitamin C and fiber.
- Always pierce a potato with a fork or knife before baking or microwaving it.
- To bake a potato, allow roughly 40 minutes at 400°F for a medium potato and an hour for a large potato. Potatoes can be baked at any temperature; simply adjust the cooking time to whatever else is in the oven. For a microwave oven, use the high setting and allow 4 minutes for a medium potato, 6 to 10 minutes for large. Cooking time will vary according to the size of the potato, the power of your oven, and the number of potatoes being cooked. Turn potato over halfway through cooking. Wrap cooked potato in a towel to let it finish cooking for 3 to 5 minutes. A potato is done if you can easily pierce it with a fork.
- Sweet potatoes can be cooked and eaten in the same manner as other potatoes.

Baked Potato Ideas:
- Mash potatoes with chicken broth and milk
- Top with a dollop of pesto or spaghetti sauce
- Top with steamed broccoli
- Serve with chili, stew, or bean or lentil soups
- Drizzle with low-fat or fat-free salad dressing
- Top with fat-free sour cream, chopped onion, and grated low-fat cheese
- Top with low-fat cottage cheese and salsa

- Mash baked sweet potatoes with brown sugar, cinnamon, and orange juice or apple cider
- Treat it like nachos: top potato with black beans, grated low-fat cheese, chopped tomatoes and jalapenos, salsa, and fat-free sour cream
- Top with fresh or dried herbs and seasonings: garlic, basil, thyme, dill, chopped chives
- Enjoy plain with salsa, ketchup, or mustard

Soup for Cyclists—There are at least four terrific things about soup. First, a pot of soup, chili, or stew goes a long way. From fridge or freezer, it makes for many simple, heat-and-eat meals. Second, except for those made with cream or cheese, soups generally are low in fat and highly nutritious. Third, soup is a tasty recovery food that can offer water, electrolytes (sodium, potassium), carbs, and protein. Fourth, you can easily cook it over a camp stove. And finally, a bowl of hearty vegetable soup is a tasty way to consume several servings of vegetables at one meal.

Canned soups and broths are a convenient alternative to homemade, and they can be just as nutritious. However, canned products generally have more sodium than homemade. Individuals on sodium-restricted diets or with high blood pressure should choose low-sodium varieties. But sweaty cyclists might welcome the added sodium after a long, hot ride.

Here are some ways to convert plain ol' canned soup into something special:

- *Combine soups:* tomato or bean + vegetable; onion + chicken noodle
- *Add ingredients:* frozen vegetables (peas, corn, carrots, spinach, broccoli); canned, diced tomato; diced chicken, cooked rice or noodles, frozen tortellini or wontons, canned, drained garbanzo or kidney beans
- *Add seasonings:* fresh herbs (chopped parsley, cilantro) or curry powder to chicken soup; cloves to tomato soup; wine, sherry or vermouth to mushroom soup; garlic powder or hot sauce to vegetable soup; cumin and chili powder to bean soup
- *Add toppings:* Parmesan cheese, grated low-fat cheese, toasted bread, or croutons

Whether you are at a campsite or your own kitchen, soup can be mmmm, mmmm good!

- **SUMMARY**—If you are like many cyclists who know what they should eat but just don't do it, you need to remember the following keys to a successful sports diet:
  - Getting too hungry is probably the biggest problem with most cyclists' diets. Good intentions to eat well easily deteriorate when cyclists get too hungry. To prevent hunger, eat appropriately sized meals on a regular schedule.
  - Plan ahead for meals and snacks. Have healthy, convenient foods available. Go grocery shopping regularly and keep your kitchen stocked.
  - Spend your calories on a variety of wholesome foods. Target at least three different kinds of food per meal and two different kinds of food per snack.
  - Enjoy hearty carbohydrate-based meals as the foundation of your cyclist's sports diet.
  - Preparing nutritious meals need not be a burden; many can be made in a matter of minutes.

Words of wisdom from other cyclists...

"Burning a lot of calories doesn't justify fueling up with a bunch of junky sugars and fats like a lot of cyclists do."
Kyla Bauer. Las Vegas, NV

"I usually spend one day a week shopping and preparing a lot of food. I cut up and wash all the fruits and vegetables, cook some chicken, and even boil and prepare pasta for the week. It saves so much time."
Kate Riedell, Fairfield, CT

"One of my favorite foods is a baked sweet potato topped with a few raisins and a little brown sugar. I pre-bake them and keep a stash in the refrigerator so I can simply reheat and eat for a snack or as part of a meal."
Louise Wilcox, Reading, MA

"I went on a group ride that started at noon so I chose not to eat lunch, fearing I wouldn't feel good riding after a meal. Big mistake! I bonked hard on some large hills. I felt lethargic, light-headed, dizzy, and definitely irritable. As soon as I finished, I devoured a turkey sub and a whole Gatorade, and I felt better. Incredible what a little food and drink can do!"
Jessica Truslow, Arlington, MA

CHAPTER 4

Vitamins and Supplements for Cyclists

VITAMINS ARE ESSENTIAL FOOD COMPONENTS THAT YOUR BODY CAN'T make. They perform important jobs, including helping to convert food into energy. Vitamins do not provide energy, however. As a hungry athlete who requires more food than the average person, you can easily consume large doses of vitamins in, let's say, a taller glass of orange juice or bigger plate of steamed broccoli. Chapter 1 has information about some of the best food sources of vitamins.

Food consumption surveys suggest that many people fail to eat a well-balanced variety of wholesome foods. Some cyclists may indeed suffer from marginal nutritional deficiencies, particularly those who restrict calories or skimp on fruits, vegetables, and dairy foods. Despite the rising popularity of supplements, most health organizations, including the American Heart Association, the American Dietetic Association, and the National Institutes of Health, recommend food, not pills, for optimal nutrition. That's because whole food is comprised of far more than just vitamins. Food contains carbohydrates, protein, phytochemicals, fiber, and other health-protective substances that are not in pills, and interact in ways that cannot necessarily be duplicated by pills. No amount of any supplement will compensate for a lousy, hit-or-miss diet and stress-filled lifestyle. Hence, the key to good health is to learn how to eat well, regardless of how busy you may be.

Vitamins and other dietary supplements are popular among athletes. Surveys suggest that 75 to 90 percent of athletes take some type of supplement with hopes it will stave off illness, enhance performance, and make them healthy. Because the Food and Drug Administration (FDA) loosely regulates dietary supplements, they can be advertised with little data proving their effectiveness or guaranteeing their safety.

Let's take a look at some of what is and is not known about dietary supplements, and then you can decide your path towards optimal nutrition.

● **FOOD FIRST**—Getting nutrients from food is first choice. Plant foods, for example, contain hundreds, perhaps thousands, of bio-active compounds called phytochemicals that provide protection against disease. The phytochemicals in colorful fruits such as tart cherries, pomegranates, blueberries, and purple grape juice may enhance recovery for muscle-damaging exercise. Of those options, purple grape juice is generally the least expensive and the most readily available at convenience stores. Drink up!

If you fail to eat well for whatever reason, supplements are an option, but it's naive to think that a pill can replace food. For example, many cyclists fail to consume a calcium-rich food at each meal, which would give them the recommended calcium intake. They may drink plenty of water and sports drinks, but not calcium-rich milk. Then they take a calcium supplement to try to compensate for this dietary oversight. While a supplement may be better than nothing, it fails to contain the whole package of nutrients found in a whole food (in this case, vitamin D, protein, potassium, and other vital nutrients).

Despite popular belief, you can get the recommended intake of nutrients by eating a variety of wholesome foods. A hungry cyclist eats more food and therefore gets more nutrients than someone who is less active and eats less. Plus, many foods that cyclists eat (breakfast cereals, energy bars) are highly fortified with extra vitamins and minerals—that is, unless you choose exclusively "all natural" options that have nothing added to them, including no extra vitamins or iron. For example, a serving of fortified cereal (Wheaties, Total) may contain 100 percent of the Daily Value (100% DV) for many vitamins and minerals, but a serving of all-natural cereal (Kashi, Puffins) may offer less than 10% DV.

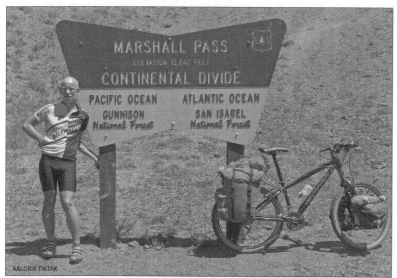

Eating a healthful, balanced diet will give your body all the nutrients it needs to perform at its best so you can achieve your cycling goals.

Cyclists Who Should Take a Supplement—Some situations put you at risk for nutritional deficiencies such as:

- *Restricting calories.* Eating less than 1,200 calories can easily result in consuming inadequate nutrients.
- *Eating a repetitive diet of bagels and pasta.* A steady diet of bagels, bread, and pasta may leave you lacking in the nutrients found in other food groups, such as iron and zinc (from meat), vitamins A and C (from fruits and vegetables), and calcium and vitamin D (from milk).
- *Skimping on fruits and vegetables.* A diet lacking fruits and vegetables is likely lacking in vitamins C and A, fiber, and antioxidants.
- *Lactose intolerance or avoidance of dairy foods.* Avoidance of dairy foods can lead to a diet deficient in calcium, vitamin D, and riboflavin.
- *Over-indulging in fats and sweets.* Filling up on nutrient-poor foods like candy and chips leaves you less hungry for healthful foods.
- *Pregnant or contemplating pregnancy.* Women require additional nutrients before and during pregnancy to help prevent birth defects. All women who may become pregnant are advised to take a multivitamin with 400 micrograms of folic

● FOR MORE INFORMATION

Confusion abounds regarding dietary supplements, their safety, and their potential health benefits. Here are some websites that offer abundant information about vitamins and health. (You might need to do a search on "vitamins" or "fish oil" to find your topic of interest):

- The American Heart Association: www.americanheart.org
- FDA's Center for Food Safety and Applied Nutrition: www.cfsan.fda.gov
- Office of Dietary Supplements: http://ods.od.nih.gov
- The World's Healthiest Foods: www.whfoods.org

For information on sports supplements, check out these websites:

- World Anti-Doping Agency: www.wada-ama.org
- National Library of Medicine: www.nlm.nih.gov/medlineplus

acid (a B-vitamin) to help prevent brain damage in the fetus. Women who are expecting should check with their physicians about which supplements they need to take.

- *Vegetarians.* People who abstain from animal products are at risk for developing B-12, iron, vitamin D, zinc, and protein deficiencies. This risk can be reduced or eliminated by choosing a well-balanced vegetarian diet.
- *Illness.* People who are sick may eat fewer calories and thus fewer nutrients, putting them at risk for deficiencies.
- *Being a senior.* Sedentary seniors require fewer calories than younger, more active adults, so they may not get all the nutrients they need.

If any of these situations applies to you, be sure to make dietary changes to enhance your food intake of the nutrients you need. Take a look at your diet to see if you are eating a variety of foods from all the food groups (grains, protein-rich foods, calcium-rich foods, fruits, vegetables). You can even track your intake at websites (such as www.fitday.com or www.sparkpeople.com) that can assess the adequacy of what you consume. Better yet, meet with a sports dietitian who can help you improve your sports diet. To find a local sports nutrition expert, use the referral network at www.SCANdpg.org.

● **IN SEARCH OF THE COMPETITIVE EDGE?**—Some cyclists look beyond simple vitamins and minerals, hoping to find sports supplements that will increase their energy, stamina, and muscle mass, and improve their athletic performance. Many sports foods, gels, or beverages are fortified with antioxidant vitamins, mega-doses of B-vitamins, herbs, caffeine, and other compounds and claim to do just that. Will these substances really give you a competitive edge? Sometimes yes, as with caffeine (see below), but generally not.

Because the FDA poorly regulates dietary supplements for quality, purity, or effectiveness, you can't be quite sure what or how much of a substance you are getting, or if (or how) it will affect you. Also consider that the sports food industry is highly competitive. Companies are adding everything from ginseng to branched-chain amino acids to their energy bars, gels, and drinks claiming it will boost performance or enhance immunity. In actuality, there is scanty scientific evidence showing these substances are helpful at all.

Below are some of the supplements of interest to many cyclists with information to help you make the appropriate decision.

B-Vitamins—Thiamin, niacin, riboflavin, pantothenic acid, biotin, B-6, B-12, and folate are referred to as B-complex vitamins. B-vitamins are essential in all metabolic and energy-producing processes in your body, and the need for B increases with intense exercise. This has led to the assumption that B supplementation will enhance energy and improve athletic performance. Scientific research does not support this assumption (Schwenk and Costley 2002).

A hungry cyclist is likely to eat more than enough B-vitamins to meet his or her requirements. Most sports supplements, foods, and drinks contain several or all of these vitamins. Grain foods such as enriched breakfast cereals, breads, and pasta are rich sources, and B-vitamins are found naturally in a wide variety of foods (nuts, meats, dried beans, lentils, vegetables, dairy foods, eggs, among others).

Caffeine—Many cyclists routinely drink a cup of coffee before they head out, saying it clears the mental cobwebs, energizes

● EAT YOUR ANTIOXIDANTS

Until science proves otherwise, your best bet for getting beta-carotene, vitamin C, and other antioxidants important for good health is to eat foods that are naturally rich in these nutrients. Use this list to guide you to an appropriate (and natural) intake of several of these health-protective nutrients.

Vitamin C: Daily Value (DV)* = 60 milligrams (mg)
The best sources include fruits (especially citrus) and vegetables.

Food	Amount	Vitamin C (mg)	%DV
Broccoli, cooked	1 cup	100	170
Orange	1	80	135
Grapefruit juice	1 cup	80	135
Kiwi	1	75	125
Cantaloupe	¼ melon	70	120

Vitamin E: Daily Value = 30 international units (IU)
The best sources are plant oils like vegetable oils and nuts. Be sure to include some of these healthful, high-fat foods in your daily calorie budget.

Food	Amount	Vitamin E (IU)	%DV
Sunflower seeds	¼ cup	12	40
Almonds	¼ cup	12	40
Wheat germ	¼ cup	7	23
Safflower oil	1 tablespoon	4.5	15
Peanut butter	2 tablespoons	4.5	15

Beta-carotene
Bright orange and yellow fruits and vegetables and dark green vegetables are rich sources of beta-carotene and other health-protective carotenoids. Beta-carotene is converted to vitamin A in the body and it is expressed as "vitamin A" on food labels. The Daily Value for vitamin A is 5,000 international units (IU).

Food	Amount	Vitamin A (IU)	%DV
Sweet potato, baked	1 medium	21,900	440
Carrot, raw	1 medium	20,250	410
Spinach, cooked	½ cup	7,400	150
Cantaloupe	¼ melon	6,880	140
Mango	1	6,420	130
Butternut/buttercup squash, boiled, mashed	½ cup	4,000	80
Romaine lettuce, shredded	1 cup	2,730	55
Broccoli, cooked	1 cup	2,415	50

1 cup = 240 milliliters; 1 tablespoon = 15 milliliters
*The Daily Value is the amount of a nutrient that meets the needs of most adults and is based on a 2,000-calorie diet.
Nutrition information from USDA National Nutrient Database (online).

them, and helps them to work harder. Caffeine's energy-enhancing effect is likely due to its ability to make exercise seem easier. Caffeine stimulates the brain and may make the effort seem easier, allowing you to work harder for longer. Once thought to have a dehydrating effect, we now know that caffeine is not dehydrating in athletes accustomed to consuming caffeinated beverages (Armstrong 2002).

If you normally abstain from coffee and caffeinated beverages, a pre-ride cup of Joe may contribute more so to a coffee-stomach and a case of the jitters than to enhanced performance. Agitation is probably the last thing you want when faced with a challenging ride or event! See chapter 9 for more information about caffeine.

Antioxidants—Beta-carotene, vitamins C and E, and selenium act as antioxidants. They deactivate destructive free radicals, compounds in the body that contribute to health problems such as heart disease and cancer. The bulk of scientific studies conclude that taking antioxidant supplements does not reduce your risk for disease. Supplementing with vitamin C, or C and E before a strenuous distance will also not reduce oxidative or immune changes (Nieman et al. 2002) or reduce muscle damage (Dawson et al. 2002). The body can handle the physical stress of intense exercise without the use of supplements. Taking too many antioxidants from supplements can actually contribute to a pro-oxidant effect that can hinder recovery. Your best bet is to eat a diet naturally rich in these nutrients—abundant fruits and vegetables.

Creatine—Creatine is a naturally occurring compound found in meat and fish. Muscles use creatine phosphate to generate energy for one to ten seconds of intense work (such as in sprinting or weightlifting). By being able to work harder, the muscles can become bigger and perform better in all-out exercise bouts (Terjung et al. 2000). Not everyone responds to supplemental creatine (Kilduff et al. 2002).

Research with racing cyclists given creatine fails to show performance improvements. The cyclists performed intervals of sprinting inserted into and at the end of a long ride. Their performance was similar with or without creatine (Hickner 2010).

The research to date suggests no physical harm from creatine if it is taken in the recommended doses. The American College of Sports Medicine advises against the use of creatine in growing adolescents; youth cyclists need to work on developing their cycling skills and learn what their body can do without supplemental creatine. As with all dietary supplements, creatine is not regulated for quality, and what you buy may not be what you get.

Ginseng—Ginseng is a plant that has been used medicinally for thousands of years in China, Japan, and Korea. Some believe that ginseng boosts mood and energy, decreases cardiovascular disease, improves athletic performance, and even acts as an aphrodisiac. These claims have yet to be supported scientifically. Most of the studies on ginseng have been poorly controlled, offer conflicting results, and are difficult to interpret. There are no good studies that support the use of ginseng for any purpose, including improving or enhancing athletic performance.

Protein supplements—Protein supplements are very popular with cyclists, yet few cyclists need supplemental protein; they consume more than enough protein via food. Excess protein does not build muscle (exercise builds muscle). Excess protein can easily displace the carbs needed to fuel muscle-building exercise. Please refer to chapter 6 for detailed information.

• **VITAMINS FOR FATIGUE**—Some cyclists complain of chronic fatigue. They feel run-down, dragged-out, and overwhelmingly exhausted. If this sounds familiar, you may wonder if a vitamin pill or other dietary supplement would solve the problem.

Perhaps you can relate to Jim, a 43-year-old long-distance cyclist. A busy, single professional, he bemoaned, "My diet is awful. I rarely eat fruits or vegetables. I live on fast foods. What vitamins should I take?" Jim lived alone and hated to cook for just himself. He rarely ate breakfast, barely ate lunch, but always collapsed after a long day with a generous fast-food feast. He struggled to wake up in the morning and stay awake during afternoon meetings. He'd grind through his training rides and gym workouts. Jim hoped some vitamins pills would restore his energy. Doubtful.

Nancy evaluated Jim's diet, calculated that he had 3,000 calories in his daily energy budget (1,000 calories per section of the day, i.e. morning, midday, evening), and suggested a few simple food changes that could result in higher energy, greater stamina, and better cycling. Nancy explored the following questions looking for solutions to Jim's fatigue. Perhaps the answers will offer solutions for your energy problems, if you have similar concerns.

- *Are you tired due to low blood sugar?* Jim skipped not only breakfast but often missed lunch because he didn't have time. He would doze off in the afternoon because he had low blood sugar. With little glucose to feed his brain, he ended up feeling sleepy. The solution was to choose to make time to eat. Just as he chose to sleep through breakfast-time, he could choose to get up five minutes earlier for breakfast. He could also choose to stop working for ten minutes to eat lunch.
- *Is your diet too low in carbohydrates?* Jim's fast but fatty food choices filled his stomach but left his muscles poorly fueled with inadequate glycogen to support his training program. Higher-carbohydrate snacks and meals would fuel his muscles and help maintain a higher blood sugar level. He'd have energy for mental work as well as physical exercise.
- *Are you iron-deficient and anemic?* Jim ate little red meat and consequently little iron, an important mineral in red blood cells that helps carry oxygen to exercising muscles. Iron-deficiency anemia can result in needless fatigue during

● THE NEED FOR SLEEP

In addition to fatigue, lack of sleep directly affects athletic performance. According to research by Peter Walters, Assistant Professor of Kinesiology at Wheaton College in Illinois, cumulative sleep deprivation has been shown to reduce cardiovascular performance by 11 percent. It also affects other measures of performances, such as focus and perceived exertion, and alters the supply of energy to the muscles. For miles of smiles, go to bed early!

exercise. Jim was taught how to boost his dietary iron intake, with or without meat (see page 64). He was referred for blood tests (hemoglobin, hematocrit, ferritin, serum iron, and total iron-binding capacity) to rule out anemia.

- *Are you getting enough sleep?* Jim's complaint about being chronically tired was justified because he was tired both mentally (from his intense job) and physically (from his strenuous training). He worked from 8 a.m. to 8 p.m. If he didn't ride at lunchtime, he'd ride or head to the gym after work. By the time he got home, ate dinner, and unwound, midnight had rolled around. The wake-up bell at 6:30 a.m. would come all too soon, especially since he often had trouble falling asleep due to having eaten such a large dinner. Nancy encouraged Jim to try to get more sleep by eating lighter dinners, such as soup and a sandwich, or cereal. He could accomplish this by eating a bigger breakfast and eating his main meal at lunch (lower-fat Chinese meals, turkey subs, chili, or pasta). By trading in 1,200 of his evening calories for 600 more calories at breakfast and 600 more calories at lunch, he could spend less time preparing and eating dinner at night. He could eat less and hopefully get to sleep earlier and with a less-full stomach.

- *Are you overtraining?* Jim took pride in the fact that he had not missed a day of training in three years, yet he felt discouraged he wasn't improving despite harder training. Nancy questioned whether he was a compulsive exerciser who punished his body or a serious cyclist who trained wisely and took rest days. One or two rest days or easy days per week are an essential part of a training program; they allow time for the body to replenish its depleted muscle glycogen.

- *Are you stressed or depressed?* Jim not only had a stressful job but was also dealing with the stress and depression associated with family problems, to say nothing of the challenges of training. Since he was feeling a bit helpless with this situation, Nancy encouraged him to successfully control and take pride in at least one aspect of his life: his diet. Simple dietary improvements would help him feel physically and mentally better about himself. This would be very energizing in itself.

If you can answer 'yes' to many of the previous questions, you may be able to resolve your fatigue with better eating, sleeping, and training habits, not with supplements. Simply experiment with the food suggestions in this book and you will transform your current low-energy patterns into a food plan for success.

● SUMMARY—

- Most cyclists can consume all the vitamins and minerals and other nutrients needed for good health by eating a variety of foods from all of the food groups.
- Extra vitamins and minerals do not enhance performance, increase energy, improve strength and endurance, or lend a competitive edge if you are already adequately nourished and suffer no nutritional deficiencies.
- By eating hearty and healthful cyclist's portions on a regular schedule throughout the day, you'll consume the vitamins, minerals, and calories you need to fight fatigue and support your exercise program.
- Protein supplements on top of an adequate diet will not improve muscle strength or size.
- Remember that dietary and sports supplements are not well-studied, are not regulated for purity and dosage, lack scientific evidence to prove their effectiveness, and most often will not improve your athletic performance. If you want more information about supplements, check out reputable websites such as Office of Dietary Supplements: http://ods.od.nih.gov.

Words of wisdom from other cyclists...

"I have always felt that eating right is the best way to get all nutrients. With my caloric intake and the variety of foods I eat, I should be fine."
Ed Kross, Framingham, MA

"I prefer to get my vitamins and minerals from foods, but just to make sure I am not missing anything, I take a multivitamin."
MaryAnn Martinez, Concord, MA

CHAPTER 5

Carbohydrates: The Fundamental Fuel

AS A SERIOUS CYCLIST, CARBOHYDRATES SHOULD BE THE FOUNDATION of each meal and snack in your sports diet. Carbs get stored in your muscles for fuel; this fuel is called muscle glycogen. When your muscle glycogen stores are low, you'll experience extreme fatigue. Carbs also travel in your blood (called blood glucose or blood sugar) and supply fuel for your brain. When your blood glucose drops, you brain lacks the fuel it needs to focus and concentrate on the task at hand. This also contributes to extreme fatigue.

You can consume carbohydrates by eating fruits, vegetables, grains, and any form of starch or sugar, be it pasta, potato, honey, sports drink, hard candy, and even marshmallows! Obviously, the best choices for good health are the "quality carbs" from fruits, vegetables, and whole grains; these give you health protective nutrients that sugary foods like candy and sports drinks fail to offer.

Today, questions abound about the role of carbohydrates in the sports diet. The purpose of this chapter is to address carbohydrate confusion and provide some clarity for cyclists who want to eat wisely for good health, weight control, and top performance.

How much carbohydrate should I eat?

Research with athletes suggests:

- The average recreational cyclist who rides an hour or so and has moderate calorie needs should target about 2 to 3 grams carb per pound body weight (5 to 7 g carb/kg). This means:

Recreational Cyclist

If you weigh:	Target grams carb/day:	Target grams carbs/meal: (Breakfast, Lunch, Lunch #2, Dinner)
100 lbs (45 kg)	200 to 300 g	50 to 75 g
125 lbs (57 kg)	250 to 375 g	60 to 95 g
150 lbs (68 kg)	300 to 450 g	80 to 110 g
175 lbs (80 kg)	350 to 525 g	90 to 130 g

- The serious racing cyclist with high calorie needs due to double workouts and exhausting high intensity rides should target about 4 to 5 grams of carb per pound body weight (8 to 10 g carb/kg). This means if you weigh 120 pounds (55 kg), you should target about 500 to 600 g carb (2,000 to 2,400 calories of carb) per day. That's a lot of pasta and bananas!

Competitive Cyclist

If you weigh:	Target grams carb/day:	Target grams carbs/meal: (Breakfast, Lunch, Lunch #2, Dinner)
100 lbs (45 kg)	400 to 500 g	100 to 125 g
125 lbs (57 kg)	500 to 625 g	125 to 155 g
150 lbs (68 kg)	600 to 750 g	150 to 185 g
175 lbs (80 kg)	700 to 875 g	175 to 220 g

To consume that much carbohydrate, recreational and competitive cyclists alike need to eat carbs as the foundation of every meal and snack: cereal for breakfast; sandwiches made with hearty

● SAMPLE 50-GRAM CARBOHYDRATE CHOICES

Here are some examples of what 50 grams of carbohydrate looks like. To consume enough carbs, make them the foundation of each meal and snack.

- Wheaties, 2 cups (60 g)
- Nature Valley Granola Bar, 2 packets (4 bars)
- Thomas' Bagel, 1 (3.5 oz)
- Banana, 2 medium
- Orange juice, 16 ounces (480 ml)
- Apple, 2 medium
- Raisins, ½ cup (75 g)
- Pepperidge Farm multi-grain bread, 2.5 slices
- Baked potato, 1 large (6.5 ounces)
- Pasta, 1 cup cooked (140 g)
- Rice, 1 cup cooked (175 g)
- Fig Newtons, 5
- Flavored yogurt + 3 graham cracker squares

breads for lunch; bananas and bagels for snacks; and pasta for dinner. The benefit will be better-fueled muscles that enable you to:
- perform with greater intensity.
- cover more distance.
- delay fatigue.

Aren't carbs fattening? Shouldn't I eat less of them so I can be leaner and lighter?

No! Carbohydrates are not inherently fattening. Excess calories are fattening. Excess calories of carbohydrates (bread, bagels, pasta) are actually less fattening than are excess calories of fat (butter, mayonnaise, oils) because the body burns energy converting excess carbohydrates into body fat. In comparison, the body easily converts excess dietary fat into body fat. This means if you are destined to be gluttonous but want to suffer the least weight gain, you might want to indulge in (high-carb) frozen yogurt instead of (high-fat) gourmet ice cream.

If carbs aren't fattening, why do high-protein diets "work"?

High-protein diets seemingly "work" because:
1. The dieter loses water weight. Carbs hold water in the muscles. For each ounce of carbohydrate you store as glycogen, your body simultaneously stores about three ounces of water. When you exercise, your body burns the glycogen and releases the water so you lose (water) weight. That's why the next time you eat carbohydrates, such as a pasta dinner, you re-gain weight quickly (you've simply reloaded your body with glycogen).
2. People eliminate calories when they stop eating carbohydrates. For example, you might eliminate not only the baked potato (200 calories) but also two pats of butter (100 calories) on top of the potato, eliminating 300 calories from your diet helps to create a calorie deficit.
3. Protein tends to be more satiating than carbohydrate. That is, protein (or fat) lingers longer in the stomach than does carbohydrate. Having 200 calories from three protein-rich eggs for breakfast satiates you longer than 200 calories from two slices of high-carb toast with jam. By curbing hunger, you have fewer urges to eat and can more easily restrict calories—that is, until you start to crave carbs and overeat

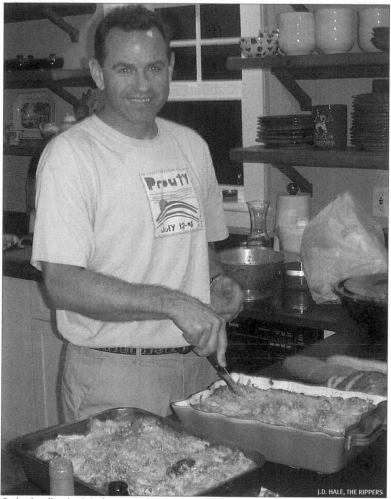
Carbo-loading both before and after events fuels-up and refuels muscles.

J.D. HALE, THE RIPPERS

them. (You know the scene: "Last chance to eat bread before I go back on my diet, so I'd better eat the whole loaf now...")

The overwhelming reason why high protein diets do not work is people fail to stay on them forever. Remember: You should never start a food program you do not want to maintain for the rest of your life. Do you really want never to eat breads, potato or crackers ever again? Your better option is to learn how to manage carbs, not avoid them. As an athlete you need carbs: Low-carb diets impair your athletic performance, prevent you from eating a balanced diet, and send the message that normal eating is "not okay."

CARBOHYDRATES: THE FUNDAMENTAL FUEL

Is there a difference between the carbohydrate from starchy foods like bread or potato versus those from sugary foods like fruit or candy?

As far as your muscles are concerned, there is no difference between sugary carbs and starchy carbs. You can carbo-load on gummy bears, bananas, or brown rice equally well. The sugar in jellybeans is a simple compound, one or two sugar molecules linked together. The starch in rice or potato is a complex compound with hundreds to thousands of sugar molecules linked together. Your muscles don't care if you eat the simple sugars or more complex starches. Both get digested and broken down into glucose, the fundamental building block of all carbohydrate. Glucose can be stored as glycogen in your liver and muscles and is used for fuel by the brain.

The difference between sugars and starches is their nutritional value and impact on health. For example, the sugar in orange juice is accompanied by vitamin C, folate, and potassium whereas the sugar in orange soda pop is void of vitamins and minerals; that's why soda is described as "empty calories." The starch in whole-wheat bread is accompanied by fiber and health-protective phytochemicals; the starch in white breads has lost its fiber and many other nutrients during the refining process.

Is white bread "poison"?

White bread offers lackluster nutrition but it is not "poison" nor a "bad" food. White bread and other refined flour products can be balanced into an overall wholesome diet, if desired. That is, if you have whole-grain cereal for breakfast and brown rice for dinner, your diet can accommodate a sandwich made with white bread for lunch. The 2010 U.S. Dietary Guidelines encourage us to consume at least half of our grain choices as whole grains. Though they pale in comparison to whole-grain products, foods made from refined flour do tend to be enriched with B-vitamins, iron, and folate, important nutrients for cyclists.

Is sugar "evil"?

Sugar is fuel, not evil. While the sugar in oranges and other fruits is accompanied by important vitamins and minerals, the sugar in, for example, candy or soda, is void of nutritional value. In general, active cyclists should limit their refined sugar

Besides rice (brown is preferable, since it has more fiber and nutritional value than white rice), try other grain varieties, such as quinoa (pronounced "KEEN-wah," a grain that contains more protein other grains), barley, millet, couscous, buckwheat, bulgur, etc. Cook a large amount to have leftovers. Here are some great ideas for your grains:

- Sweet grains: Add dried cranberries, raisins, dates, or apricots when grains are done but still steaming to plump them up.
- Add nuts or seeds such as sunflower seeds, pine nuts, or chopped pecans.
- Make a grain loaf or burgers: Combine cooked grains with eggs, reduced-fat cheese, ground nuts or seeds, or cooked lentils or beans. Then shape into burgers or a loaf and bake.
- Make a grain-based salad: Combine cooked grain, hot or cold, with any and all vegetables and a little of your favorite dressing.
- Toss in feta or other (reduced-fat) cheese.
- Use leftover cooked grains to make breakfast porridge. Add milk and cook until soft. Sweeten with fruit, raisins, and/or honey or brown sugar.

intake to about 10 percent of total daily calories. That's about 250 to 300 calories of sugar per day, roughly 48 ounces of Gatorade (two large bike bottles), two to three sports gels, 20-oz bottle of soda pop, or 15 to 20 gummy bears.

Most athletes can handle sugar just fine. But for a few, sugar seems "evil" because it contributes to swings in blood sugar levels (hypoglycemia, or low blood sugar) that can result in feeling lightheaded and shaky. If you are sensitive to sugar and notice that eating sugar makes you feel bad, eat some protein with it, such as peanut butter with jelly in a sandwich, low-fat cheese with an apple, a glass of milk with fig cookies, or almonds with raisins.

Note that sugar taken *during* exercise is unlikely to contribute to a hypoglycemic reaction because muscles quickly use the sugar without the need for extra insulin. This includes sports drinks, gels, sports beans, gummy candies, and other popular sugary choices. (See chapter 10 for more advice about pre-exercise fueling.)

Should I avoid eating sugar before my workouts?

Unless you are sensitive to sugar as noted in the previous question, there is no reason to avoid it prior to exercise if it fits into your overall balanced diet. However, craving sugar before an afternoon ride can be a sign that you have gotten too hungry. You can prevent the cravings for sugary, quick-energy foods by eating a bigger breakfast and lunch(es). The best advice regarding pre-exercise sugar is to avoid the desire for it by eating heartier meals prior to exercise.

Should I choose foods based on their glycemic effect?

Not necessarily. The glycemic effect of a food refers to the rate at which the food raises blood sugar. Also called "glycemic index," it is a non-exact science. That's because a body's reaction to a food varies from person to person and from meal to meal, and also depends on the combinations and quantity of foods eaten. Rather than rely on the glycemic index, you should experiment with a variety of high-carbohydrate foods like grains, fruits, and vegetables to learn what food combinations settle well for you, satisfy your appetite, and offer lasting energy.

What are some examples of carb-based meals?

As a serious cyclist, you may be unable to get adequate carbs from just fruits and veggies to fuel your muscles. So be sure to include some pasta, potato, rice, or other starch in your meal menu. Here are a few suggestions:

- *Breakfast:* raisin bran, Grape-Nuts and other cold cereals, granola, oatmeal, bagels, muffins, pancakes, waffles, English muffins, toast, French toast
- *Lunch:* sandwiches made on hearty wholesome breads; hearty soups with beans, lentils, pasta; vegetable pizza with thick crust
- *Dinner:* meals with pasta, potato, rice, noodles, or other grains covering most of the plate; extra vegetables; rolls
- *Snacks* (and accompaniments to meals): fruit juice, bananas, fruit smoothie, dried fruit, pretzels, baked chips, fig cookies, flavored yogurt, frozen yogurt, hot cocoa/chocolate milk

Be sure also to include some protein as an accompaniment to the carbs. While carbs fuel the muscles, protein builds and repairs muscles. The next chapter offers more details about the right balance of carbs and protein. Keep reading!

• SUMMARY—

- Carbohydrates should not be a source of confusion. To the contrary: Wholesome carbs—fruits, vegetables, and grains—clearly should be the foundation of your sports diet. You need them to fuel your muscles so you can be strong throughout your ride, day after day.

- As a dedicated cyclist, you may be unable to get adequate carbs from fruits and veggies alone, so be sure to include some pasta, potato, rice or other starch in your meal menu.

- If desired, enjoy refined carbohydrates, like soda pop, sugar, and sports drinks, in moderation (less than 10% of daily calories).

- By "carbo-loading" every day, your muscles will have the fuel they need to train at their best. This will help you enjoy mile after mile, recover quickly, and feel good.

Words of wisdom from other cyclists... ━━━━━━━━━━━━━

"I like to cook Japanese sticky rice* with a little salt, make it into balls, and store them in baggies. They are really good on longer rides— a nice break from the sweet stuff."
(**Sticky rice Is short-grain or "sushi" rice and comes brown or white.*)
Marcia Gibbs, California

"On long rides, I bring sweet potatoes— I bake them and carry two in my pocket."
Rich Lesnik, San Francisco, CA

"I microwave small red potatoes, wrap them in plastic after salting, and eat them on long bike rides. I get tired of sweet things and these really hit the spot, provide energy, and fill me up."
Ruth Carey, Portland, OR

CHAPTER 6

Protein for Muscles

BETWEEN ADS FOR PROTEIN SUPPLEMENTS AND THE FALSE RUMORS about carbs being fattening, many cyclists wrongly think protein should be the foundation of their sports diets. They believe if they eat a lot of protein, they will build a lot of muscle. If that were true, we could simply devour large portions of meat and end up looking quite buff!

Eating excess protein offers no benefits to a sports diet. The extra protein you eat does not turn into extra muscle; it is either burned for energy or stored as fat. A balanced sports diet plus resistance exercise—in the form of lifting weights or pushing hard on pedals when you are grinding up a steep hill—is what builds muscle. Fueling your muscles with wholesome carbohydrates, not excessive amounts of protein, assures you will have enough energy to perform muscle-building exercise.

You need adequate protein, about 10 to 15 percent of your day's calories, to build and repair muscles, make red blood cells, enzymes, and hormones, and allow hair and fingernails to grow. This translates into a small-to-medium portion of protein at each carbohydrate-based meal.

Eating too little protein leads to chronic fatigue, anemia, lack of athletic improvement, muscle wasting, poor healing, and an overall run-down feeling. Iron and zinc deficiencies can occur with a protein-poor diet, since they are primarily found in protein-rich foods. Cyclists at risk of protein deficiency include vegetarians who don't eat enough nuts, beans, and plant proteins, and long-distance cyclists who eat too many bagels and bananas but not enough meat or dairy food.

- **HOW MUCH PROTEIN IS ENOUGH?**—*How to Balance Your Protein Intake* on page 60 can help you calculate your protein needs and compare it to what you actually consume.

The protein recommendation of 0.5 to 0.8 grams per pound of body weight (1.2 to 1.7 g/kg) is based on these assumptions:
- You are eating plenty of calories. Your protein needs increase if you are dieting.
- Your muscles are well-fueled with carbohydrates. You burn more protein for fuel if your muscles are glycogen-depleted. Most cyclists and other athletes typically consume more than the recommended protein intake.

To meet your protein needs, include a serving of protein-rich food as an accompaniment to each carbohydrate-based meal. The following menu gives a sample day with approximately 100 grams of protein, more than enough for a 160-pound cyclist.
- *Breakfast:* 8 ounces low-fat milk (9 grams protein) on cereal
- *Snack:* 2 tablespoons peanut butter (8 grams protein) on bread
- *Lunch:* 4 ounces turkey and 1 slice of cheese (30 + 6 grams protein) in a sandwich
- *Snack:* 8 ounces low-fat yogurt (8 grams protein)
- *Dinner:* 4 ounces meatballs (30 grams protein) with pasta and ½ cup kidney beans (7 grams protein) on a salad

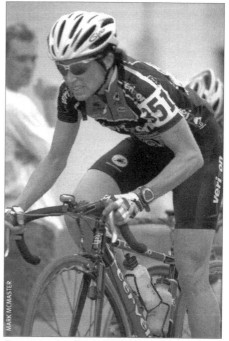

Most grains and starchy vegetables provide 2 to 3 grams of protein per serving. So this menu actually provides more protein than indicated.

Note how quickly the grams add up from animal proteins. Four ounces of cooked meat, chicken, or fish is roughly the size of a deck of playing cards and has 25 to 30 grams of protein. Plant proteins can provide a lot of protein too, if you eat enough of them. If you eat only a little peanut butter (2 tablespoons has only 8 grams of protein) on a lunchtime

To get to the finish line, you need adequate protein as well as abundant carbohydrates.

● HOW TO BALANCE YOUR PROTEIN INTAKE

If you wonder if you are eating the right amount of protein, you can estimate your daily protein needs by multiplying your weight by 0.5 to 0.9 grams of protein per pound (1.1 to 2.0 grams of protein per kilogram).

Daily Protein Requirements

	Grams of protein per pound of body weight	Grams of protein if you weigh:		
		120 lb	150 lb	180 lb
RDA for sedentary adult	0.4	50	60	70
Recreational cyclist, adult	0.5-0.7	60-85	75-105	90-125
Endurance cyclist, adult	0.6-0.7	70-85	90-105	110-125
Growing teenage athlete	0.7-0.9	85-110	105-135	125-160
Cyclist building muscle mass	0.7-0.8	85-95	105-120	125-145
Cyclist restricting calories	0.8-0.9	95-110	120-135	145-160
Maximum required for adults	0.9	110	135	160

Use food labels and the following chart to calculate your protein intake. Pay close attention to portion sizes!

Protein Content of Some Commonly Eaten Foods

Food	Protein (g)	Food	Protein (g)
Tuna, 1 can (6.5 ounces)	40	Pasta, 2 ounces dry, or 1 cup cooked	8
Chicken or turkey breast, roasted, 4 ounces	35	Oatmeal, ½ cup dry, or 1 cup cooked	6
Beef, pork, cooked, 4 ounces	30	Rice, ⅓ cup dry, or 1 cup cooked	4
Salmon, cooked, 4 ounces	30	Cold cereal, 1 ounce	2-3
Egg, 1 large	7	Bread, 1 slice	2
Egg white, from 1 large egg	3	Potato, white or sweet, 1 small, baked w/skin	2-3
Soynuts, ¼ cup roasted	16	Peas, ½ cup cooked	4
Tofu, raw, firm, ½ cup cubes	10		
Peanut butter, 2 tablespoons	8		

Food   **Protein (g)**
- Almonds, 1 ounce (24 nuts) — 6
- Black beans, ½ cup — 7
- Hummus, ½ cup — 6
- Soymilk, 1 cup — 5-7
- Milk, 1 cup — 8-10
- Yogurt, 1 cup — 8-10
- Cheddar cheese, 1 ounce — 8
- Cottage cheese, ½ cup — 14

Fruits, non-starchy vegetables

Most fruits and vegetables have negligible amounts of protein. They may contribute a total of five to ten grams of protein per day, depending on how much of them you eat.

Nutrition information from food labels, USDA National Nutrient Database (online), and J. Pennington, 2004, Bowes & Church's Food Values of Portions Commonly Used, 18th ed. (Philadelphia: Lippincott, Williams & Wilkins)

1 cup = 240 milliliters;
1 tablespoon = 15 milliliters; 1 ounce = 28 grams
1 kilogram = 2.2 pounds

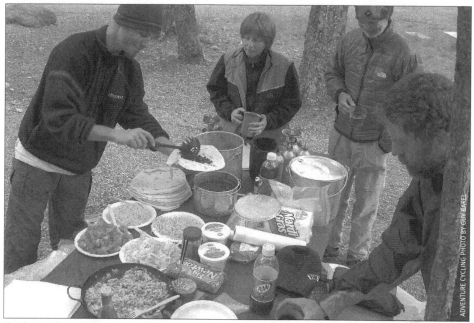

Touring cyclists prepare bean burritos at a campground. Rich in protein and carbohydrates, canned beans are a convenient alternative to meat or poultry.

sandwich and just a sprinkling of garbanzo beans (½ cup has only 7 grams protein) on a dinnertime salad, you will fall short of meeting your protein needs.

● **PROTEIN POWDERS, SHAKES, AND BARS**—Cyclists commonly believe they should consume protein shakes and protein bars to enhance their sports diet. What makes you think you need additional protein? Most hungry cyclists get more than enough protein through standard foods. When you are on the run and grabbing meals, yes, a protein shake or protein bar can be a convenient way to get hassle-free, low-fat protein. If you are touring, yes, a protein bar can be handy "emergency food." But because those are engineered foods, they lack the wholesome goodness and yet-to-be identified compounds found in all natural sources of protein. See page 89 for more information.

Carbohydrate deficiency in athletes is far more common than protein deficiency! Protein supplements are not only costly and needless but also displace bananas, whole-grain bagels, and other sources of carbohydrate that fuel the muscles. Don't get swayed by advertising that tries to convince you otherwise.

● **VEGETARIANS AND PROTEIN**—Vegetarians can indeed consume enough protein to build muscles and maintain health if they choose their diets carefully. The key is to eat plenty of high-protein foods that contain a variety of the essential amino acids, the building blocks your body requires for making and maintaining muscle. Animal sources of protein (meat, fish, poultry, eggs, and milk) offer complete protein. That is, they contain a good balance of all of the essential amino acids. Plant proteins (grains, nuts, soy, and legumes) have limited amounts of some of these amino acids. Someone who eats no animal proteins (a vegan) must therefore eat a variety of plant proteins to get sufficient amounts of all the essential amino acids.

● **TIPS FOR MEAT EATERS**—Red meats, such as beef, pork, veal, and lamb, present a dilemma for many cyclists. Meat is an excellent source of protein. It is rich in iron and zinc, two minerals necessary for optimal health and athletic performance. On the other hand, meat contributes saturated fat and cholesterol to the diet, and it presents ethical and environmental concerns. If you choose to eat red meat, select lean cuts of meat and eat them in moderation. Chicken, turkey, and fish have less saturated fat and are heart-healthier options.

Animals and all food products derived from them contain cholesterol. Generally speaking, most animal proteins, chicken and fish included, have similar cholesterol values: 70 to 80 milligrams of cholesterol per four-ounce serving. The American Heart Association recommends that healthy people with normal blood cholesterol levels consume less than 300 milligrams of cholesterol per day. Small portions of red meat can certainly fit those requirements.

In terms of heart health, the cholesterol content of meat is of less concern than the saturated fat content. Fatty meats such as greasy hamburgers, pepperoni, juicy steaks, and sausage are poor choices but are often the easy option for touring cyclists who stop at local diners. Lean meats, such as London broil, extra-lean ground beef, top-round roast beef, lean ham, pork loin, turkey breast, and roasted or grilled chicken, provide less saturated fat and are better choices for a healthy sports diet. See chapter 7 for more information on fat and cholesterol.

Here a few ideas to help you with a meat-free diet that has adequate protein.

Breakfast:
- Cold cereal (preferably iron-enriched, as noted on the label): Add milk, yogurt, or soymilk, and sprinkle with a few nuts.
- Oatmeal, oat bran, and other hot cereals: Add peanut butter, almonds or other nuts, and/or powdered milk.
- Toast, bagels: Top with low-fat cheese, cottage cheese, or peanut butter.

Snacks:
- Assorted nuts
- Peanut butter on rice cakes or crackers
- Yogurt (Note: Frozen yogurt has only 4 grams of protein per cup, as compared to 8 grams of protein per cup of regular yogurt and 20 grams per cup of Greek yogurt.)

Lunch and Dinner:
- *Salads:* Add tofu, tempeh, chickpeas, three-bean salad, marinated kidney beans, low-fat cottage cheese, sunflower seeds, chopped nuts.
- *Protein-rich salad dressing:* Add salad seasonings to plain yogurt, blenderized tofu, or cottage cheese (diluted with milk or yogurt).
- *Spaghetti sauce:* Add diced tofu, or canned, drained kidney beans.
- *Pasta:* Choose protein-enriched pastas that offer 13 grams of protein per cup (as compared to 8 grams per cup of regular pasta). Top with grated part-skim mozzarella cheese.
- *Potato:* Bake or microwave, then top with canned beans, baked beans, or low-fat cottage cheese.
- *Hearty soups:* Choose lentil, split pea, bean, and minestrone.
- *Hummus:* Try hummus with pita or tortillas.
- *Cheese pizza:* Half of a 12-inch pizza has about 40 grams of protein.
- *Burrito:* Top a flour or corn tortilla with canned refried beans and low-fat cheese.
- *Vegetarian burgers and dogs:* Try a soy "hamburger" patty or "hotdog" on a whole-grain bun.

Iron—Red meat is arguably one of the best dietary sources of iron for two reasons:

1. Red meat contains more iron per ounce than fish or poultry.
2. The iron in animal protein, known as heme-iron, is absorbed more easily than the iron from plant sources.

● HOW TO BOOST YOUR IRON INTAKE

- The recommended intake for iron is 8 milligrams for men and 18 milligrams for women per day. Women have higher iron needs to replace the iron lost from menstrual bleeding. Women who are post-menopausal require only 8 milligrams of iron per day.
- Iron from animal products is absorbed better than that from plant products.
- A source of vitamin C at each meal enhances iron absorption.

Animal Sources (best absorbed)	Iron (mg)	Vegetables	Iron (mg)
		Spinach, ½ cup cooked	3
Beef liver, 4 ounces cooked	7	Broccoli, ½ cup cooked	1
Beef, 4 ounces cooked	3	**Beans**	
Shrimp, 4 ounces cooked	4	Kidney beans, ½ cup cooked	3
Chicken leg, 4 ounces cooked	2	Tofu cubes, ½ cup	3
Pork, 4 ounces cooked	1	**Grains**	
Chicken breast, 4 ounces cooked	1	Cereal, 100% iron fortified, 1 cup	18
Salmon, 4 ounces cooked	1	Spaghetti, 1 cup cooked	2
Egg, 1 large	1	Bread, enriched, 1 slice	1
Fruits		**Other**	
Prunes, 5	1	Molasses, blackstrap, 1 tablespoon	3
Raisins, ⅓ cup	1		
Dried apricots, ⅓ cup	1	Wheat germ, ¼ cup	2

1 cup = 240 milliliters; 1 tablespoon = 15 milliliters; 1 ounce = 28 grams; 4 ounces = 112 grams
Nutrition information from food labels, USDA National Nutrient Database (online), and J. Pennington, 2004, Bowes &
Church's Food Values of Portions Commonly Used, 18th ed. (Philadelphia: Lippincott, Williams & Wilkins)

Failure to consume adequate iron can lead to anemia, a chronic depletion of iron-rich red blood cells that will leave you weak, tired, vulnerable to illness, and unable to perform at your best. Women, who lose iron through monthly menstrual blood losses, are at high risk for becoming anemic. A routine blood test can rule-out that possibility.

Zinc—Ordinarily, foods rich in iron are also rich in zinc, and red meat is no exception. If you don't eat meat or if you eat an iron-poor diet, chances are your diet is lacking in zinc. Zinc is important for healing minor, day-to-day tissue damage as well as major injuries and ailments. Like iron, the zinc in red meat and other animal protein is better absorbed than the zinc in plant foods or supplements. For non-meat eaters, particularly those who do not eat fortified breakfast cereals, a multi-vitamin/mineral pill with both zinc and iron can help supplement the diet.

Poultry: Chicken, Turkey, and Eggs—If you do not eat red meats, you might want to include more dark meat from chicken or turkey in your sports diet to get more iron and zinc. The darker meats include the wings and drumstick (leg + thigh). These cuts do contain more fat relative to white breast meat, but they also supply more minerals. The skin on chicken and turkey is mostly fat and lacks nutrients, so it is wise to peel it off before or after cooking and discard it.

Eggs are an excellent, inexpensive source of high-quality protein. Egg whites are mostly water with 3 grams of protein per egg. The nutrient-dense yolk adds another 3 grams of protein, along with polyunsaturated fat and about 185 milligrams cholesterol. (The American Heart Association recommended consuming less than 300 milligrams cholesterol per day.) No longer shunned for their cholesterol content, eggs are accepted to be part of a heart-healthy sports diet. As with all foods, moderation and variety are key, so enjoy some eggs each week, if you like, preferably poached or cooked with olive or canola oil.

Get Hooked on Fish—Protein-rich seafood can be a rich source of omega-3 fat, the good fat that protects against cardiovascular disease: heart attacks, narrowing arteries, and strokes. You're never too fit nor too young to consider a heart-healthy diet. Cyclists are not immune from heart disease, and early signs of the disease appear in children as young as age 12! The American Heart Association recommends eating two fish meals per week, particularly oily fish, such as trout, salmon, sardines, and herring.

If you avoid fish because you are concerned about contaminates such as mercury and PCBs (polychlorinated biphenyls), it may help you to know that the health benefits of eating fish generally far outweigh the risks. The trick to eating fish wisely is to avoid the fish which are known to be high in mercury, such as king mackerel, shark, and swordfish, and to consume a variety of other fish. For instance, choose two different kinds of seafood each week (or better yet, six to eight different kinds per month) from these recommended fish: arctic char, catfish, tilapia, sardines, herring, halibut, cod, pollock, haddock, trout, salmon (canned or wild Alaskan), yellowfin or canned light tuna, and shellfish like oysters, scallops, mussels, and clams. Baked, broiled, seared (with little or no oil), or steamed are the healthiest ways to enjoy seafood. The grease in fried fish can negate the healthfulness of the fish.

● SUMMARY—

- Protein should be an *accompaniment* to every sports meal, not the main focus.
- Low-fat milk, yogurt, fish, eggs, poultry, and meats are protein-rich choices; beans, nuts, lentils, and soy products provide protein in smaller amounts. If you prefer a vegetarian diet, plan to have a protein-rich plant food with each meal.
- "Vegetarians" who simply eliminate meat but make no effort to include alternate plant sources of protein, iron, and zinc can suffer from dietary deficiencies that hurt their sports performance and their health.
- Contrary to popular notion, eating a lot of protein does not enhance muscle growth, strength, or size. The best way to build muscle and strength is through resistance training and a wholesome, carbohydrate-rich diet.

- While lean red meat can be a nutrient-dense sports food, the *saturated fat* in greasy red meats, not the red meat itself, is the primary health culprit. Poultry and fish are lower in saturated fat. Fish has the added benefit of providing heart-healthy omega-3 polyunsaturated fat.
- Protein bars should be used only as "emergency food" when you are eating on the run and your protein needs would otherwise be neglected.

Words of wisdom from other cyclists... ━━━━━━━━━━━━━━━━

"I tend to eat a vegan diet for personal reasons, but have learned over the years to listen to my body and if on occasion I really crave steak, well, I have it."
MaryAnn Martinez, Concord, MA

"I'm a semi-vegetarian. I get my 'protein fix' by eating a lot of beans, lentils, and tofu, along with Greek yogurt, milk, nuts, and cheese."
Elizabeth, Massachusetts

"As a vegetarian, I incorporate protein into each meal. For example, I eat almond butter on whole-grain toast for breakfast. I add seitan, tempeh, or tofu to stir-frys, soy crumbles to chili or spaghetti sauce, and enjoy various types of beans with quinoa or brown rice for lunches and dinners."
Kathy Martin, Massachusetts

CHAPTER 7

Fats and Your Sports Diet

Eat fat, get fat. Eat fat, clog your arteries.
Eat fat, have a heart attack. Eat fat, pedal slow.

YOU'VE PROBABLY HEARD THIS ANTI-FAT CHATTER. WHILE THERE IS AN element of truth in some of these statements, there is also room for more education. Let's look at the whole picture.

While all dietary fat used to be considered bad, we now know that all fats are not created equal.

- The hard, saturated fat in greasy meats, red meat, butter, and cheese is the "bad" fat that is associated with high blood cholesterol levels, cardiovascular disease, and even cancer.

- Considered "very bad fat" is trans-fat, the hydrogenated and partially hydrogenated fats in some commercial foods, such as stick margarine, pie crust, bakery items like muffins, cookies, and cakes, and deep-fat fry oils. These are considered to be worse for your health than saturated fats.

- The soft, liquid polyunsaturated and monounsaturated fats in fish, avocados, olives, liquid vegetable oils, peanuts, seeds, and nuts are the "good" fats, essential for fighting inflammation and heart disease, and investing in overall good health. Olive oil, the foundation of the heart-healthy Mediterranean Diet, is health-protective. For centuries native Italians and Greeks have enjoyed good health and meals with about 40 percent of the calories from fat.

There's no need to avoid all fat like the plague. A little, preferably "good," fat at each meal helps you to absorb certain vitamins (A,D,E,K), provides essential fatty acids, may improve athletic performance by reducing inflammation, and gives you greater satiety and satisfaction from meals. Plus long-distance cyclists who include some fat in their daily training diet are more likely to enjoy greater stamina and endurance than those who try to exclude fat.

Whereas a little bit of fat is an appropriate part of a sports diet, too much fat is not:

- A high-fat diet can displace carbohydrates, leaving your muscles unfueled.
- Fat has over twice the calories of protein or carbohydrate, so excess fat calories can add up easily and lead to weight gain.

Cyclists who eat too much fat would do better to substitute some of their fat calories for more carbohydrates. Carbs replace depleted muscle glycogen stores; fats do not.

- **HOW MUCH FAT SHOULD YOU EAT?**—Most healthy cyclists can target a sports diet with about 25 percent of the calories from fat. This amount of fat:

- is consistent with the 20 to 35 percent fat diet that is considered to be health-protective;
- gives you enough carbohydrates (55 to 65 percent of total calories) for restoring muscle glycogen and enough protein (10 to 15 percent of total calories) for muscle maintenance and repair;
- allows for easier participation in life (i.e., eating at a party, enjoying a cookie guilt-free); and
- gives you enough fat for taste and good nutrition without providing excess calories that contribute to weight gain.

How does 25 percent fat translate into food? Let's say you have 2,400 calories a day in your calorie budget (this would be a reducing diet for a 160-pound recreational cyclist who wants to lose excess body fat):

0.25 x 2,400 total calories = 600 calories a day of fat.
Because there are 9 calories per gram of fat,
divide 600 calories by 9:
600 calories ÷ 9 calories per gram = 66 grams of fat
in your daily fat budget.

High-mileage cyclists may need 3,500-5,000 calories a day. That allows space for more fat grams. To estimate your daily calorie budget, see chapter 15.

A 25-percent-fat diet includes a reasonable amount of fat

● FAT GUIDELINES

The following guidelines can help you appropriately include fat in your food plan.

Calories per day	Fat grams per day (for a 25% fat diet)
1,800	50
2,000	55
2,200	60
2,400	65
2,600	70
2,800	75
3,000	85

Fat and Calories in Common Foods

Food	Amount	Fat (g)	Cal.	Food	Amount	Fat (g)	Cal.
Milk products				Ice cream, gourmet	½ cup	15	250
Milk, whole (3½% fat)	1 cup	8	150	Ice cream, light	½ cup	3	110
				Frozen yogurt, low-fat	½ cup	2	120
Milk, low-fat (1%, ½% fat)	1 cup	2	100	**Animal proteins (cooked weight)**			
Milk, fat-free	1 cup	—	80	Beef, hamburger	4 oz.	24	330
Cheddar cheese	1 oz.	9	110	Top sirloin	4 oz.	10	240
Cheddar cheese, reduced-fat	1 oz.	5	90	Chicken breast, no skin	4 oz.	5	200
Cottage cheese (4% fat)	½ cup	5	120	Chicken thigh, no skin	4 oz.	11	235
Cottage cheese, low-fat (2% fat)	½ cup	2	90	Haddock	4 oz.	1	125
Cream cheese	2 T	10	100	Swordfish	4 oz.	6	175
Cream cheese, light	2 T	5	60	**Fruits and vegetables**			
				most varieties		negligible fat	

and lets you enjoy a little fat at each meal. Preferably you'll choose the good fats which have positive health value. If you hanker for the occasional big burger (with 25 grams of fat and 500 calories), be sure to balance it into your day's fat and calorie budget and optimize the rest of the day's meals. But be aware that all fats are not created equal. That burger or ice cream splurge is saturated fat and is not the same as splurging on a jar of peanuts or a bowl of guacamole (avocado) which is unsaturated fat. Try to swap foods rich in "bad fat" with those that contain more "good fats" (see page 72). See the guidelines for fat in the above chart to estimate how many fat grams you should target per day.

Fat and Calories in Common Foods

Food	Amount	Fat (g)	Cal.	Food	Amount	Fat (g)	Cal.
Vegetable proteins				Spaghetti, cooked	1 cup	1	210
Beans, kidney cooked	½ cup	—	110	Rice, cooked	1 cup	—	200
Tofu	4 oz.	5	90	**Fast foods**			
Peanut butter	1 T	8	95	Big Mac	1	30	570
Mixed nuts	1 oz. or 3 T	15	170	Egg McMuffin	1	12	290
Fats				French fries	small	10	210
				Fried chicken	1 breast	24	400
Butter, Margarine	1 T	12	105	Pizza, cheese	1 slice	10-13	250
Oil, olive	1 T	13	120	**Snacks, treats**			
Mayonnaise	1 T	11	100	Cookie, Chips Ahoy	1	2	50
Grains				Fig Newton	1	1	60
Bread, large slice whole wheat	1	1	90	Brownie	1 small	5	140
Saltines	5	2	60	Graham crackers	2 squares	1	60
Ritz	4	4	70	Potato chips	18 (1 oz.)	9	150
Rice cake, large	1	—	35	Pretzels	1 oz.	1	110
Shredded wheat	1 oz.	—	90	Milky Way	1.75-oz. bar	8	220
Granola	1 oz.	6	130	M&Ms with peanuts	1.75-oz. bag	13	250
Oatmeal, uncooked	1 oz.	2	100				

1 cup = 240 milliliters; 1 tablespoon (T) = 15 milliliters; 1 oz. = 28 g = 28 ml; 4 ounces = 112 grams

Nutrition information from food labels, USDA National Nutrient Database (online), and J. Pennington, 2004, Bowes & Church's Food Values of Portions Commonly Used, 18th ed. (Philadelphia: Lippincott, Williams & Wilkins)

● **FEAR OF FAT**—Without a doubt, fat imparts a tempting taste, texture, and aroma and helps make food delicious. That's why fatty foods can be hard to resist and are often enjoyed to excess. Although excess calories from fat can easily turn into body fat, the eat-fat-get-fat theory is false. What does add to body fat is eating excess calories—not just from fat but also from protein, carbohydrate, and alcohol. Many cyclists eat appropriate amounts of fat and stay thin. They simply don't overeat total daily calories.

If you are weight-conscious and obsess about every gram of fat to the extent you have a fat phobia, your fear of fat is exaggerated. A little fat can actually aid in weight reduction. Dietary fat contributes to the nice feeling of being satisfied after a meal, and may help you eat less during and after a meal. For example, you may have less desire to keep munching on, let's say, yet another cracker if you start by eating a cracker with a little peanut butter. Refer to the weight reduction information in chapter 16 for additional help with resolving your eat-fat-get-fat fears.

As mentioned before, you want to include a little fat in each meal not only to help absorb certain vitamins for optimal health but also to enhance performance. In a study with runners, those who boosted their intake of healthful fat from 17 percent of calories to 30 percent of calories were able to run longer and also had less inflammation afterwards. Inflammation contributes to muscle fatigue and damage.

Meal	Instead of these (rich in saturated or trans fat):	Choose these (rich in mono- and/or poly-unsaturated fat):
Breakfast	Croissant	Bagel with peanut butter
	Cheese omelet	Vegetable omelet
	Donut	Whole-wheat toast with almond butter
	Muffin	Handful of cereal with raisins and nuts added
Lunch	Roast beef sandwich	Peanut butter sandwich
	Turkey and cheese sub	Tuna sub made with reduced-fat mayonnaise
	Roll-up with cheese, veggies	Roll-up with hummus, veggies
	Cheese on a salad or sandwich	Avocado or olives on a salad or sandwich
	Bologna, salami	Canned sardines or tuna
Snack	Cheese, full-fat	Almonds or olives
	Packaged cookies or chocolate	Dried fruit and nut mix
Dinner	Blue cheese salad dressing	Vinaigrette or Italian dressing
	Butter on a roll	Olive oil on a roll
	Steak	Grilled fish
	Fettuccine with alfredo sauce	Fettuccine with garlic, olive oil
	Spaghetti with meatballs	Spaghetti with clam sauce
	Hamburger	Veggie or salmon burger
	Vanilla ice cream	Low-fat frozen yogurt sprinkled with nuts

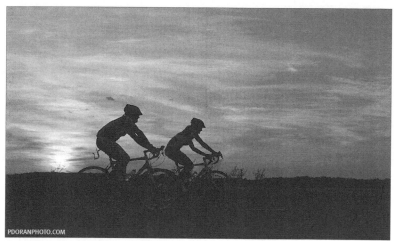

A sports diet with healthful fat enhances endurance, handy when the ride lasts longer than anticipated.

• SUMMARY—

- All fats eaten in moderation can be balanced into an overall healthful and carbohydrate-based sports diet.
- Cyclists who include some fat in their daily sports diet are able to perform better than those who try to exclude fat.
- Eating too much fat can lead to poorly fueled muscles, excess calories, and weight gain.
- Choosing more of the healthful fats—olive oil, canola oil, nuts, avocado, fish—is preferable to loading up on the fat from butter, cookies, greasy burgers, and ice cream.

Words of wisdom from other cyclists... ▬▬▬▬▬▬▬

*"As a general rule, I try to avoid most high-fat meals.
I'm not afraid of fat, just aware of when and what kind I am eating.
The majority of my fat intake comes from natural peanut butter
(either in smoothies or sandwiches), olive or sesame oil in my rice or
pasta dishes, and avocado (sprinkled with salt and pepper)."*
Ryan Fletcher, Denver, CO

CHAPTER 8

Fluids, Water, and Sports Drinks

DEHYDRATION IS ONE OF THE MAJOR CAUSES OF FATIGUE WHILE BIKING long distances. Hence preventing dehydration is a vital part of your sports diet. Recreational cyclists who ride for an hour or less in cool weather are unlikely to become dehydrated. Long-distance and/or racing cyclists who pedal hard for longer need to be more careful, even in cool weather (but especially in hot weather). They might be losing one to two quarts (liters) of fluid per hour, if not more. With repeated days of riding, that really adds up.

During hard exercise, your muscles can generate 15 to 20 times more heat than they do when you are at rest. To dissipate the heat and keep the body from overheating, you release sweat. Evaporating sweat cools your skin. This in turn cools the blood and reduces your body temperature. Some cyclists sweat profusely, soaking their helmets and riding jerseys even on shorter rides. Others seem to barely sweat at all. In dry climates and cold weather, you may not feel like you sweat as much, but you still lose fluids while exercising. All cyclists in all climates in all seasons need to be attentive to replacing sweat losses.

● **HOW MUCH SHOULD YOU DRINK?**—For optimal hydration, you should balance your fluid losses with your fluid intake as you go along. To determine how much fluid you lose while biking, your "sweat rate," weigh yourself naked before and after one hour of riding without eating or drinking. For every pound you lost, you shed 16 ounces of sweat.

When biking in the heat, pay attention to your buddies and also listen to your own body. If you notice that you or your friends feel light-headed, dizzy, nauseated, clumsy, uncoordinated, confused, irrational, have stopped sweating, or have ashen gray pale skin, stop biking immediately! These are all symptoms of heat illness.

Here's what to do:
• lie down in a shady or cool place
• raise legs and hips to improve blood pressure
• remove excess clothing
• cool off by wetting the skin liberally and fanning vigorously
• if possible, apply ice pack to groin, armpits and neck
• drink cool water

Many cyclists make the mistake of waiting until they are thirsty to drink. Bad plan. When you reach this point you are already dehydrated. By the time your brain signals thirst you may have lost 1 percent or more of your body weight. Your goal should be to limit sweat loss to 2 percent of your body weight (ACSM 2007). That is,

If you weigh:	Do not lose more than:
100 lbs (45 kg)	2.0 lbs (1.0 kg)
125 lbs (57 kg)	2.5 lbs (1.2 kg)
150 lbs (68 kg)	3.0 lbs (1.5 kg)
175 lbs (80 kg)	3.5 lbs (1.6 kg)

Your heart rate increases by 3 to 5 beats per minute for every 1 percent of body weight loss. With increasing sweat losses, exercise feels harder, you'll enjoy it less, and you'll pedal slower. In extreme cases becoming dehydrated can contribute to medical problems.

When you ride hard day after day in the heat you can easily become chronically dehydrated. You'll feel unusually fatigued and lethargic. Don't let that happen!

You can tell if you are well hydrated by monitoring your urine:
• You should urinate every 2 to 4 hours throughout the day.
• The urine should be pale colored and of significant quantity. (Your urine may be dark yellow if you take multivitamin supplements. In this case, volume of urine is a better indicator of hydration than is color.)
• Your morning urine should not be scanty and concentrated.

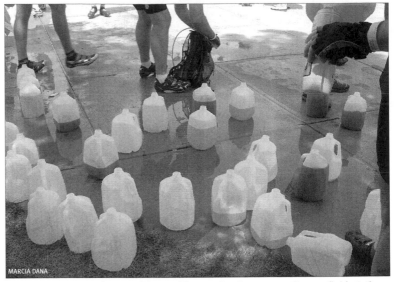

At the Pan-Mass challenge, riders refill water bottles at one of many fluid stations. Depending on your sweat rate, you should plan to drink about one large bike bottle (24 ounces) per hour during a ride.

Since the sensation of thirst can be an unreliable indicator to drink, you should program your drinking according to your sweat rate. Drink on a schedule so that you do not fall short of your fluid goals. For example, drink four gulps (roughly 4 ounces or 120 milliliters) every 15 minutes. Practice drinking during training rides to become familiar with the skills involved in drinking while riding as well as your body's capacity for fluids. When you get off the bike, drink enough to quench your thirst plus more just to be safe.

● **ELECTROLYTE REPLACEMENT**—When you sweat, you lose electrolytes, such as sodium and potassium, two of the minerals that help maintain proper water balance in your tissues. Contrary to what many athletes think, commercial sports drinks include these electrolytes *not* to replace those lost in sweat but primarily to enhance retention of water in your body. Most cyclists who ride or race for a couple of hours do not have to worry about replacing electrolytes during exercise because the losses are generally too small to cause a deficit that will hurt performance and/or health.

But for exercise that lasts four hours or more, occurs in very hot weather, or goes on for several days (randonnée, tour,

THE CYCLIST'S FOOD GUIDE: FUELING FOR THE DISTANCE

The average male's body contains about 75,000 milligrams of sodium, the amount found in 11 tablespoons (200 grams) of salt. While you may lose some sodium when you are riding, you are unlikely to deplete your body's supply. In an hour of riding you may lose 400 to 1,500 milligrams, depending on:

How much you sweat. On cooler days where you sweat little, you won't lose as much sodium.

How much you exercise in the heat and how fit you are. If you are fit and acclimatized to hot weather, you will conserve sodium to defend against sodium depletion.

stage race) electrolyte losses can become problematic, particularly if you are consuming little more than plain water during that time. Drinking too much plain water during extended, sweaty exercise can create an electrolyte imbalance in your body. In particular, a low level of sodium in the body, or hyponatremia, causes fatigue, nausea, headache, cramps, and diarrhea. If left unchecked, hyponatremia can lead to confusion, poor coordination, seizures, and even death.

If you plan to ride hard for more than four hours, plan to consume sodium and potassium during the ride, such as found in bagels, bananas, tomato or V-8 juice, pretzels, salted nuts, broth, ham & cheese sandwiches, oatmeal raisin cookies, and endurance sports drinks. If you're on a ride that lasts for several days, be extra careful to include salty foods in your daily meal plan, for example, salt in your morning oatmeal, mustard on your lunchtime sandwich, and soup or tomato sauce with dinner. If you crave salt, you likely should eat some salty foods. See *Comparing Fluid Replacers* on page 78.

● **SPORTS DRINKS OR WATER?**—During rides that last longer than 60 to 90 minutes, you will perform better if you consume more than just plain water, particularly if you are not going to be eating solid food. Sports drinks are a convenient way to consume small amounts of carbohydrates to fuel your mind and muscles, and a little sodium and potassium to enhance water retention. But keep in mind, most sports drinks are essentially just sugar water with a dash of salt.

A pound of sweat contains on average 100 milligrams of potassium and 400 milligrams of sodium. In two hours of sweaty riding, you might burn at least 1,200 calories and lose 64 ounces (2 liters) of water, 400 milligrams of potassium, and 1,600 milligrams of sodium in your sweat. To help you recover these losses, you can choose from these popular options.

Per 8 oz/240 ml

Fluid	Calories	Carb. (g)	Sodium (mg)	Potassium (mg)
Water	0	0	0	0
Vitamin Water	50	13	0	0
Gatorade	50	14	110	30
Powerade	70	19	55	30
Cytomax	70	15	75	80
Accelerade	90	17	125	40
Cola	100	25	5	—
Beer	100	7	12	60
Light beer	65	3	6	40
Orange juice	110	25	2	475
Cranberry-apple juice drink	165	40	5	65
Low-fat milk	100	12	125	380
Chocolate low-fat milk	160	25	150	425
V8 juice	50	10	420	470
Fruit yogurt (low-fat)	225	40	120	450

Nutrition information from food labels, product websites, and J. Pennington, 2004, Bowes & Church's Food Values of Portions Commonly Used, 18th ed. (Philadelphia: Lippincott, Williams & Wilkins)

If you consume food during a ride, such as pretzels and salted nuts, or muffin and juice, those foods can do the job of replacing carbohydrates and electrolytes. There's no need for a sports drink; you'll be fine hydrating with plain water.

If you are riding hard, you may prefer to drink your calories rather than eat solid food. That's when a sports drink can be helpful. Experiment with a variety of brands and flavors of sports drinks to determine which ones you prefer to drink. That will be the best choice for your body!

● **HOW TO KEEP YOUR COOL**—Here's a short true-false quiz to test your knowledge about fluid replacement and help you survive the heat in good health and with high energy

Despite popular belief, salt for athletes is not a four-letter word. The public health recommendations to reduce salt intake are directed to people who are overweight, under-fit, and have high blood pressure, not lean, fit cyclists with normal or low blood pressure.

How much salt do cyclists actually need?

Salt (or more correctly sodium, the part of salt that is the health culprit) requirements depend upon how much you sweat. A "safe and adequate" sodium intake for the average person is 2,300 milligrams per day. The typical American intake is 3,000 to 6,000 milligrams of sodium per day, which tends to cover the sodium needs of most cyclists.

- The rule of thumb is to add extra salt to your diet if you have lost more than four to six pounds of sweat (3 to 4 percent of your body weight pre- to post-ride).
- Too little salt can result in fatigue and muscle cramps.
- Cyclists and other athletes who sweat profusely day after day and eat primarily low-salt foods may benefit from adding a little sodium to replace that lost in sweat.
- If you'll be riding for longer than four hours, drink and/or eat foods that contain added salt, such as sodium-containing sports drinks, pretzels, deli meats (in a sandwich), vegetable juices, soups, and energy bars.

True or False: Drinking cold water during exercise will cool you off.

True, but only by a small margin. Drinking cold water will cool you off slightly more than warmer water, but the difference is small because the water quickly warms to body temperature. The more important concern is quantity. Any fluid of any temperature is better than no fluid.

Cold fluids tend to be more palatable than warm fluids, hence are the more popular option. In hot weather, when fluids left on the bike become warm, consider freezing drinks first and then drink them as they thaw, and/or invest in a thermal water bottle or covering.

True or False: Weight-conscious cyclists should pay attention to liquid calories.

True. The calories you drink are more likely to contribute to fat gain than calories you chew. That's because liquid calories

● SODIUM-RICH PORTABLE SNACK FOODS

If you are one of the many cyclists who thinks you need to buy a sports drink to replace the sodium you lose in sweat, think again. Sodium-rich portable sports snacks can easily fit into a backpack or handlebar bag and provide more sodium than most commercial sports drinks. These salty suggestions can be a welcome flavor change if you have been downing sweet gels, sports candies, and sugary drinks for several hours.

Portable Snack	Amount	Sodium (mg)	Calories
Gatorade	8 oz. (240 ml)	110	50
Triscuits	1 oz. (5 crackers)	180	120
Salted Peanuts	1 oz. packet	190	170
Pretzel Nibblers, Snyder's	1 oz. (16)	200	120
Ritz Bits	1 oz. packet	230	140
Clif Mojo Sweet & Salty Trail Mix Bar	1 bar	230	200
Wheat Thins	1 oz. (14 crackers)	200	120
Bagel	½ medium	270	150
Saltine crackers	1 oz. (10 crackers)	300	120
Pretzel-Thin Twists, Snyder's	1 oz. (11 twists)	330	110
V8 Juice	Small (5.5 oz) can	330	30
Red Oval Stoned What Thins	1 oz. (4 crackers)	420	120
Pretzel sticks, Bachman	1 oz. packet	520	100
Beef jerky, Jack Link's	1 oz.	590	80
Boiled potato + ¼ tsp salt	1 medium	600	150
Pretzel Rod, Rold Gold	1 rod (1 oz.)	610	110
Chicken Bouillon cube, Herb-Ox	1 cube	1100	5

Information from food labels, May 2011; 1 oz. = 28 grams

are less filling and don't contribute much to satiety (that nice feeling of having been fed). Think of a regular soda as a sugary treat, not as a water alternative.

True or False: Drinking water 30 minutes before exercise eliminates the need to drink fluids during a long training session.

False. Research suggests that drinking a quart of water before exercise is less effective than drinking an equal volume during exercise. Researchers aren't sure why, but they recommend the optimal approach: Tank up beforehand plus drink enough to match your sweat losses during exercise.

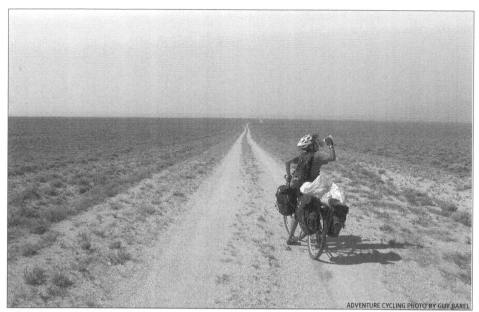

When you are faced with a long road ahead of you and no known water source, tank up beforehand, carry extra water, and take frequent water stops.

True or False: Don't bother to drink during a ride that is shorter than an hour because the fluid has too little time to get into your system.

False. According to Larry Armstrong, exercise physiologist at the University of Connecticut, water can travel from stomach to skin in just 9 to 18 minutes after drinking. This water is essential for dissipating the heat you produce during exercise. Your best bet is to try to match sweat losses with an equal volume of fluid intake during exercise, even if it's under an hour.

True or False: Beer is an appropriate recovery fluid.

False. Although beer is a popular recovery drink, it lacks what your depleted body needs after exercise. Beer and most other alcoholic beverages are poor sources of the carbohydrates needed to refuel your muscles: A 12-ounce (360-milliliter) can of beer has only 14 grams of carbohydrates. The same amount of juice or soft drink has 40 grams.

Alcohol has a dehydrating effect, and it acts as a depressant. If you drink alcohol on an empty stomach, as commonly happens post-race, you can quickly negate the pleasurable "natural high" that you would otherwise enjoy.

FLUIDS, WATER, AND SPORTS DRINKS |

● MUSCLE CRAMPS

Muscle cramping during exercise can occur in both super-fit cyclists and beginners. There are two separate causes for muscle cramping in healthy cyclists:

1. Muscle fatigue
Exhaustive cycling can lead to cramps in overworked and unfit muscle(s). This cramping is not related to electrolyte or sodium losses.

2. Excessive sweating
High sweat losses and consequent sodium deficiency can lead to widespread muscle cramping. Sometime called "exertional heat-cramps," these can occur in either cold or hot environments where there is extensive sweat loss.

To reduce your risk of cramping
- Consume enough salt and fluid during exercise to offset your sweat/sodium losses.
- If you are a heavy sweater, be conscientious and ingest high-sodium foods during long bouts of cycling.

Note: Sweat losses of potassium, magnesium, and calcium are unlikely causes of muscle cramping.

Wise beer-drinkers first have one or two glasses of water and eat some carbohydrate-rich foods (pretzels, baked chips, crackers), and then they enjoy a beer or two in moderation. Alternatively, they skip the beer and enjoy chocolate milk—an excellent recovery beverage! (For more information on post-ride recovery, see chapter 12.)

● SUMMARY—

- Cyclists who fail to drink enough fluid on a daily basis will suffer from chronic fatigue.
- Your best bet is to prevent dehydration by drinking enough fluid throughout the day, so that you need to urinate every two to four hours and your urine is pale colored.
- Do not overhydrate. Excess fluid can dilute sodium levels, lead to hyponatremia (low blood sodium), and cause serious medical problems.
- Drinking a sports drink during an extended ride can be an easy way to consume carbohydrates and sodium as well as

water. Cyclists who eat food while riding can appropriately drink plain water.

- The standard sports diet provides more than enough sodium, but if you crave salt or are a salty sweater, you likely should eat some salty foods to replace sodium lost in sweat.

Words of wisdom from other cyclists... ━━━━━━━━━━━━━━━━━

*"Biking in Houston, Texas, can be very hot and humid!
I like to pre-freeze bottles of sports drinks or water for the ride.
They thaw quickly when it's so hot outside and
the chilled beverage tastes better."*
Paula Mrowczynski-Hernandez, Houston, TX

*"I'm very diligent about keeping myself hydrated...
there's nothing worse than crossing the finish line with
the driest tongue stuck to your mouth!"*
Kate Riedell, Fairfield, CT

*"On long, hot rides, I have done a dual Camelbak approach
where I put water in one bladder and a sports drink in the other."*
Doug Davis, Dallas, TX

*"For long rides, I drink orange juice and tomato juice,
which I can get on the road at convenience stores.
These have lots of potassium and the tomato juice has sodium,
which help me feel better on a ride."*
Rich Taylor, Concord, MA

*"I work with people who do ultra-distance riding in the Texas heat.
As the riders gradually increase their ride lengths, we weigh them
before and after each ride. We match the water weight lost with fluid intake.
By the time the 250-mile days come around, our riders know how much
they should consume along the way. It's interesting to watch people
realize that they really do have to drink more than they thought."*
Doug Davis, Dallas, TX

CHAPTER 9

Commercial Sports Foods: Convenience or Necessity?

TO LOOK AT ALL THE ADS FOR SPORTS DRINKS, ENERGY BARS, ELEC-trolyte replacers, and sports candies, you'd think these engineered products are a necessary part of a sports diet. Both recreational and competitive cyclists commonly ask for advice about how to use these products. Many cyclists believe commercial sports foods are the best sources of carbohydrates and electrolytes. Wrong. In most cases, a wisely chosen sports diet can supply all your needs—plus more!

While there is a time and a place for commercial sports foods (particularly among racing cyclists who train at high intensity), many touring and recreational cyclists needlessly waste a lot of money misusing them. The purpose of this chapter is to help you become an informed consumer, so you can wisely spend your food dollars.

● **PRE-EXERCISE ENERGY BARS**—Fueling with an energy bar and sports drink is an expensive way ($2 to $3) to energize your workout. You could less expensively consume 300 calories of banana + yogurt + water ($1) or pretzels + raisins + water ($.50). Any of these choices is carbohydrate-rich and will offer the fuel your muscles need for a stellar workout. Commercial energy bars do not contain any magic ingredients that will enhance performance more than, for example, a granola bar, bagel, or fig cookies and water. Standard supermarket foods can do that as well as engineered foods.

● ENERGY BARS: WHICH ONE IS BEST?

Some energy bars are glorified cookies, while others are wholesome snacks. If you frequently consume energy bars, choose the wholesome ones. They are all rich in carbs that fuel your muscles. So choose the bar that tastes best to you and settles well.

- **All-natural/organic** (have no added vitamins or minerals): Clif Bar, Peak Energy, Perfect 10, Clif Nectar, Clif Mojo, Lara Bar, Optimum, TrailMix HoneyBar, Odwalla Bar, PowerBar Nut Naturals, Honey Stinger Bars, Kashi Bars
- **Granola-type bars:** PowerBar Harvest, Nature Valley Granola Bar, Quaker Chewy Bars, Nutri-Grain Bar
- **Women's bars** (have fewer calories and contain soy, calcium, iron, and folic acid): PowerBar Pria, Amino Vital Fit, Luna Bar, Balance Oasis
- **40-30-30 Bars** (40% carb, 30% protein, 30% fat): Balance Bar, ZonePerfect
- **Kosher:** Pure Fit, Lara Bar, Extend Bar, Raw Revolution
- **Dairy-free:** Clif Nectar, Pure Fit, Perfect 10, Lara Bar, Clif Builder's Bar
- **Gluten-free:** Perfect 10, Elev8Me, Hammer Bar, Clif Nectar, EnvirKids Rice Cereal Bar, Omega Smart Bars, Odwalla Bar, Clif Builder's Bar, Extend Bar, Zing Bar
- **Fructose-free:** JayBar
- **Vegan:** Pure Fit, Lara Bar, Hammer Bar, Vega Whole Food Raw Energy Bar, Clif Builder's Bar, Perfect 10, Raw Revolution
- **Bars with caffeine:** Peak Energy Plus
- **Vitamin & protein-pumped candy bar:** Marathon Bar, Detour Bar
- **Recovery bar** (3 or 4:1 carb:protein ratio): PowerBar Recovery

The best pre-ride snacks digest easily, settle well in your stomach, and do not "talk back to you." Experiment to determine what foods your body accommodates best. Refer to chapter 10 for more information about how to fuel before exercise.

● **ENERGY DRINKS**—Energy drinks such as Red Bull and Full Throttle offer enough sugar and caffeine to give most any athlete a quick energy boost. The problem is, one quick fix will not compensate for missed meals. That is, if you sleep through breakfast and barely eat lunch, having a Red Bull for a pre-workout energizer will unlikely compensate for the previous inadequate food

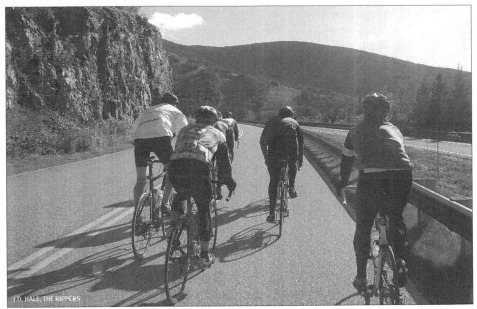
When riding in a pack, commercial sports foods can be an easy and convenient way to stay fueled.

intake. If you can make the time to train, you can also make the time to fuel appropriately, rather than rely on a quick fix.

Caffeine—A popular "ergogenic aid," caffeine enhances performance by making the effort seem easier. Cyclists who are accustomed to consuming caffeine can energize their workout by consuming caffeine pre-exercise, especially if they also consume carbohydrates (such as a bagel or banana). But for other cyclists, caffeine can make them feel nervous, jittery, and nauseated. Be sure to experiment with pre-exercise caffeine during training to determine how your body responds. In general, an effective intake is about 1.5 mg caffeine per pound of body weight (3 mg/kg), or about 200 mg for a 130-pound cyclist.

Here's how the options compare:

Option	Caffeine	Cost
Black tea, brewed 1 bag	55 mg	$0.10
Coca-Cola, 20 oz.	60 mg	$1.59
Red Bull, 8 oz.	80 mg	$2.19
No-doz, 1 tablet	200 mg	$0.33
Coffee, home brew, 16 oz.	200 mg	$0.20
Starbuck's coffee, 16 oz.	350 mg	$1.95

At one time, caffeine was thought to have a dehydrating effect, but that is not true. Research suggests caffeine does not contribute to excessive water loss and is okay to consume, even in the heat (Armstrong 2002, 2005).

● **SPORTS DRINKS**—Many athletes believe the sodium in sports drinks is essential to replace the sodium lost in sweat. Wrong. Sports drinks are actually relatively low in sodium compared to what you consume in your meals. As discussed in chapter 8, sodium enhances fluid retention and helps keep you better hydrated, as compared to plain water.

Despite popular belief, there is no need for any cyclist to consume a sports drink with their lunch because the soup or cheese sandwich offers far more sodium than the small amount of sodium in the sports drink. By consuming some salty food such as 8 ounces of chicken broth before riding in the heat, you can get a hefty dose of sodium into your body before you even begin to ride. This has also been shown to enhance endurance (Sims 2007).

Electrolytes—Some cyclists drink sports drinks all day, thinking the beverage is important to replace electrolytes—and then may admit they don't even know what electrolytes are! Electrolytes are electrically charged particles and include (among others) sodium, calcium, magnesium, and potassium. Standard foods abound with these electrolytes, more so than engineered sports foods. Note how few electrolytes the engineered foods contain compared to standard foods:

	Sodium	*Calcium*	*Magnesium*	*Potassium*
Endurolytes (1 capsule)	40 mg	50 mg	25 mg	25 mg
Hammer Gel	25 mg	—	—	25 mg
HEED, 1 scoop	40 mg	51 mg	26 mg	25 mg
Nuun, 1 tab	360 mg	12 mg	25 mg	100 mg
Peanut-butter & jelly sandwich & milk	600 mg	300 mg	130 mg	750 mg
PowerBar Blasts (1 pouch)	60 mg	—	—	—
Pizza, 1 slice (⅛ of 12-inch)	650 mg	200 mg	20 mg	160 mg

Homemade Sports Drink

The nutritional profile of commercial sports drinks is 50 to 70 calories per 8 ounces (240 milliliters), with about 110 milligrams sodium. Below is a simple recipe that offers this profile, but at a much lower cost than the expensive store-bought brands. You can make it without the lemon juice, but the flavor will be weaker.

You can be creative when making your own sports drink. For example, you can dilute many combinations of juices (such as cranberry + lemonade) to 50 calories per 8 ounces and then add a pinch of salt. (More precisely, ¼ teaspoon salt per 1 quart of liquid.) Some people use flavorings such as sugar-free lemonade to enhance the flavor yet leave the calories in the range of 50 to 70 calories per 8-ounce. The trick is to always test the recipe during training, not during an important event. You want to be sure it tastes good when you are hot and sweaty and settles well when you're working hard.

¼ cup sugar (50 g)

¼ teaspoon salt (1.0 g)

¼ cup hot water (60 ml)

¼ cup orange juice (60 ml) not concentrate, plus 2 tablespoons (30 ml) lemon juice

3½ cups cold water (840 ml)

1. In the bottom of a pitcher, dissolve the sugar and salt in the hot water.

2. Add the juice and the remaining water; chill.

3. Quench that thirst!

YIELD: **1 quart or 4 (8-oz or 240-ml) servings**
Nutrition Information per serving

CALORIES	50
CARBOHYDRATE	12 g
SODIUM	110 mg

Vitamin Waters and Vitamin-Enriched Sports Foods—Many sports beverages tout they are enriched with B-vitamins "for energy." True, B-vitamins are needed to convert food into energy, but they are not sources of energy. The body has a supply of vitamins stored in the liver, so you are unlikely to become deficient during exercise.

Cyclists—who eat far more food, hence more vitamins, than do sedentary people—have the opportunity to consume abundant vitamins. A large bowl of Wheaties offers 100% of the Daily Value (DV) for B-vitamins. Most cereals, breads, pastas, and other grain foods are enriched with B-vitamins. ("All-natural" grains, however, have no vitamins added to them.)

Eight ounces (240 milliliters) of orange juice offers 100% DV for Vitamin C. In contrast, 8 ounces of Energy Tropical Citrus Vitamin Water offers only 40% DV for C. Check labels on all these products to comparison shop.

• **SPORTS GELS AND SPORTS CANDY**—During intense rides, consuming a gel, sports drink, or sports candy can help boost your energy. So can any sugary food: honey, jellybeans, defizzed cola.

Think twice before you spend your money on, let's say, Sport Beans ($1 for a 100-calorie packet) for an off-bike afternoon snack. Like sports drinks and gels, Sport Beans are designed to be consumed *during* exercise. Regular jellybeans would be a far less expensive snack. Better yet, raisins, dried pineapple, or a banana is a healthier snack option. See chapter 11 for more information about fueling during rides.

• **PROTEIN POWDERS, AMINO ACIDS, AND BRANCHED-CHAIN AMINO ACIDS**—Protein is made up of amino acids, the building blocks of protein. There are 21 amino acids. Your body can manufacture all but nine of the amino acids. These are referred to as "essential" amino acids because you must consume them in your diet. When you eat chicken, nuts, eggs, and any protein-rich-food, your body breaks down the protein into amino acids. The amino acids circulate through the blood, and if needed, they are recombined to build various tissues in the body. If you overeat protein, the extra amino acids are burned for energy or stored as fat.

Taking extra amino acids will not help your performance. To date, no scientific evidence indicates that individual amino acids have a bodybuilding, performance-enhancing, or immune-stimulating effect. Taking a protein supplement on top of an adequate diet (0.5 gram of protein per pound of body weight, or 1.0 gram per kilogram) will not enhance muscle strength or size (Godard, Williamson et al. 2002).

Three of the essential amino acids, isoleucine, leucine, and valine, are called branched-chain amino acids (BCAA). These have been studied for their possible role in delaying fatigue during exercise, in part because BCAA levels decline with exercise. To date, the studies are inconclusive. Some show improved mental function or reductions in perceived exertion with supplementation of BCAA, but most do not demonstrate a positive effect on performance (Fragakis 2003). The best way to prevent the decline of BCAA during exercise and to enhance your performance is to consume carbohydrates before, during, and after exercise (Davis 1995).

The amino acids in supplements are not better than the amino acids found in naturally in protein-rich foods. You can easily get all the essential amino acids you need by eating regular food and getting adequate protein. The advantages of food include more vitamins, minerals, and other nutrients. Plus, food costs much less than supplements: A 6-ounce can of tuna costs about one dollar and provides 30 grams of protein; a PowerBar ProteinPlus costs almost double that price and provides less (24 grams) protein.

Until more research proves otherwise, your best bet for maximum performance is to get your amino acids through food. By eating protein-rich choices such as chicken, meat, fish, soy, and dairy products as part of your healthy diet, you can get more than enough protein to build and repair your muscles. See chapter 6 for more information about protein.

● SUMMARY—

- Commercial sports foods can be a convenient source of pre-wrapped calories that travel well, but they are not magic.
- Many cyclists report standard foods taste better and are more enjoyable. As an educated consumer, learn which foods work best for your body.
- Always *experiment first during training* with any new food or fuel that you might use during an important ride!

━━━━━━━━━━━━━━

"When it comes to commercial sports foods versus regular food,
I feel it is best to be a true omnivore, especially on long rides.
It dramatically increases your choices."
Elmar Stefke, Berkeley, CA

"It's important to know your fuel and how to use it.
For example, I use Clif Shot Bloks because I know exactly what each
chew contains. Plus, it is easy to grab out of my jersey pocket when navigat-
ing off-road."
Cato Coleman, Columbus, OH

"Some sports bars and gels can be super-sweet,
so I balance them with Fig Newtons, animal crackers, pretzels, and
peanut butter sandwiches on long rides."
Paula Mrowczynski-Hernandez, Houston, TX

"If I am going to ride for a while, I will have a sports gel
an hour into the ride and repeat this every hour I'm on the bike.
This combined with a bottle of sports drink per hour gives me roughly
300 calories of carbohydrates per hour and helps prevent
the downward spiral of energy depletion."
MaryAnn Martinez, Concord, MA

Fueling Before You Ride

EATING BEFORE RIDING PROMISES ADVANTAGES THAT CONTRIBUTE TO better performance, more energy and stamina, and faster recovery. But food and drink can sometimes be a problem for people who fear upset stomachs, abdominal cramps, and bathroom stops that interfere with riding. This chapter provides useful information about pre-exercise food and drink to help you devise a pre-ride nutrition strategy that will maximize your performance and enjoyment during every ride.

• **FIVE BENEFITS OF PRE-RIDE FOOD**—Research demonstrates that eating more carbohydrates (or carbo-loading) the days before an event maximizes muscle glycogen stores and improves performance in events lasting 90 minutes or more. Consuming carbohydrates three to four hours before exercise tops off liver and muscle glycogen stores and enhances endurance performance. For touring cyclists, this advantage can mean the difference between fully enjoying or barely enduring a day of riding. For competitive cyclists, it can mean the difference between a podium finish and getting dropped by the pack. Here are some helpful facts to give you some insight about the benefits of eating before riding.

The carbohydrates you eat even an hour before riding are digested and converted to glucose to:
1) top off your body's glycogen stores,
2) be used for energy by muscles, thereby sparing your glycogen stores, and thus
3) delay the onset of fatigue.

● TRAIN LOW, COMPETE HIGH?

Some cyclists "train low" (with low glycogen stores) to enhance their muscles' adaptation to burning more fat. Then, they "compete high" with fully loaded glycogen stores in hopes of burning more fat, sparing the limited glycogen, and performing better.

While this strategy can reduce the reliance on carbohydrates during exercise, there is no clear evidence that this strategy enhances performance. The present research is limited; we need more studies that mimic "real life" situations (Burke, 2010). Stay tuned!

Take note: Training with low blood glucose is hard work and not fun. It limits your ability to do quality workouts, and also can be can be dangerous if you lose focus and end up having an accident.

1. Pre-ride carbohydrates fuel the muscles.—Your body has approximately 1,800 calories worth of carbohydrates (or glucose) stored as glycogen in the muscles (1,400 calories) and liver (350 calories). These limited stores influence how long and how hard you can enjoy riding. When your muscle glycogen stores get low you "hit the wall." Your legs begin to lose power and strength; you feel exhausted and want to stop. Your performance and mood rapidly decline. By consuming adequate carbohydrates before (and during) your ride, you can delay the onset of fatigue caused by muscle glycogen depletion.

In contrast to your very limited glycogen stores, you have nearly 100,000 calories worth of fat in your body. Unfortunately for endurance cyclists, the body cannot use just fat to fuel itself; it requires carbohydrate to burn fat. Without carbohydrates your body breaks down muscle protein for energy.

2. Pre-ride food fuels the brain.—The brain requires a steady supply of glucose from glycogen stored in the liver. When liver glycogen stores are depleted, blood sugar levels drop, your brain is deprived of adequate glucose, and you suffer the effects of hypoglycemia. Referred to as "the bonk," you become lightheaded, irritable, and sleepy. You have blurred vision and are unable to think clearly to make good decisions. A poorly fueled brain also impairs muscle function and mental drive.

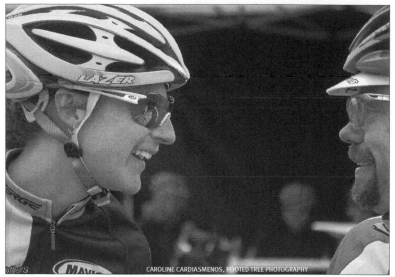

Fuel-up well before long rides to assure you and your riding partners miles of smiles.

One racer (now a pro racer and coach) once bonked so badly he got off his bike during the actual race, wandered over to some shady grass, and took a nap (obviously not only sleepy but also judgment-impaired)! To prevent the dreaded bonk and the danger that comes with it, you need both pre-ride carbohydrates and a steady supply during rides.

If you ride first thing in the morning with nothing to eat, you have essentially fasted since dinnertime the evening before and you will improve your stamina and mental drive by consuming some carbohydrates before heading out. Some early morning riders consume nothing yet report that they have plenty of energy. Most likely they ate a substantial dinner and/or serious late-night snack the night before which bolstered liver glycogen stores and reduced the need for a morning energizer. This is not bad or wrong as long as this pattern works well for them.

You want to choose the carbs that settle best and are well-tolerated. Some riders wonder if they should choose quickly absorbed, high-glycemic carbs (sugar, potato) for quick energy, or slowly absorbed, low-glycemic carbs (oatmeal, yogurt) for sustained energy. When it comes to performance, research has not consistently demonstrated a benefit from consuming low- or moderate- versus high-glycemic foods prior to exercise. Some

To be sufficiently fueled for long training rides, hard workouts, races, or all-day riding events, you should do minimal exercise the day before and plan your meals according to this schedule. Always drink additional fluids with and between meals to ensure complete hydration. If you tend to be overly nervous or have a sensitive stomach prior to a stressful event, you may want to limit your food intake on that day and make a special effort to eat extra food the day before. If you are on a bike tour, you need to wisely eat and drink throughout the day to invest in sustained energy for the length of the tour.

Morning event

Day before: Eat a hearty, high-carbohydrate lunch, dinner, and bedtime snack.

Event day: Eat a comfortable, carbohydrate-rich snack/breakfast to abate hunger feelings and get your blood glucose on the upswing.

Afternoon event

Day before: Eat a hearty, high-carbohydrate dinner.

Event day: Eat a hearty high-carbohydrate breakfast and a comfortable lunch, as tolerated.

Evening event

Event day: Eat a hearty, high-carbohydrate breakfast and lunch. Eat a comfortable, carbohydrate-rich snack 1 to 3 hours prior to the event, as tolerated.

research studies show people can exercise harder and longer with low-glycemic foods pre-exercise, and other studies do not. This may be explained by individual glycemic responses to foods. Your best bet is to experiment during training to see what works for you. For instance, if you have been eating a pre-exercise microwaved potato, try a fruit yogurt instead to see if it contributes to better performance. Keep in mind: rather than fret about what to eat before a long ride, know that fueling *during* the ride is the better way to enhance stamina and endurance.

3. Pre-ride food helps settle the stomach, absorbs some of the gastric juices, and abates hunger.—For many people, the stress associated with competition or other cycling events stimulates gastric secretions and contributes to an "acid" stomach. Eating a small amount of food can help alleviate that problem. Eating 100 to 300 calories of a low-fat, carbohydrate-rich snack within the hour before riding will provide fuel and should sit comfortably in your stomach. Try eating a small bowl of oatmeal, half a bagel, or a few crackers. You'll learn by trial and error what foods work, what foods don't.

4. Pre-ride beverages can provide fluids to fully hydrate your body as well as additional carbohydrates.—By tanking-up on sports drinks or diluted juice before you ride, you help prevent dehydration and boost your carbohydrate and energy intake. You should drink plenty of fluids every day whether you ride or not, in both hot and cold weather. Frequent urination and clear-colored urine are confirmations that you drank adequately. If your urine is dark and concentrated, you need to drink more. Refer to chapter 8 for more information on hydration.

5. Pre-ride food can pacify your mind with the knowledge that your body is well-fueled.—Before a long ride or race, you don't want to waste any energy wondering if you have eaten enough. Appropriate eating can resolve that concern! Pre-exercise food has great psychological value. If you firmly believe that a specific food will enhance your performance, then it probably will. Your mind has a powerful effect on your body's ability to perform at its best. If you have a magic food that assures athletic excellence, you should take special care to be sure it is available prior to the ride.

● **HOW MUCH TO EAT**—Because everyone is unique, it is difficult to define the optimal amount of food you should eat before heading out on the bike. Eating 200-300 grams of carbohydrate (800-1200 calories) 3 to 4 hours prior to exercise has been shown to enhance performance. Eating the hour before exercise may or may not have an effect on your performance, depending on how much you ate earlier (ACSM 2009). We know of cyclists who can eat a pile of pancakes an hour before riding and others who can barely handle juice.

What you can tolerate before and during a ride depends on many things, including how hard you will ride, the time of day, and your fitness level. The key to tolerating ride food is to experiment with food and drink during training to learn

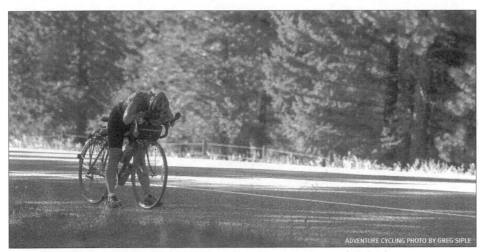

To prevent bonking, consume carbohydrate-based meals and snacks on a daily basis, and consume carbohydrates before and during your ride.

through trial and error:

- What foods and fluids work best for you, and when (that is, do you tolerate oatmeal before a recreational ride, but only sports drink before an intense hill climb?)
- What works for you at what time of day (does your usual pre-ride bagel for afternoon rides sit like a brick for morning rides?)
- When you should consume them (do you feel best eating one hour before a ride, or three?)
- How much is appropriate (simply a banana, or a banana plus a sandwich?)

● EXPERIMENTING DURING TRAINING TO KNOW WHICH BRANDS IN WHICH AMOUNTS YOU CAN TOLERATE—We emphasize *experimenting during training* because here is what typically happens. Cyclists read advertisements or hear fellow cyclists talking about special sports drinks, energy bars, gels, supplements, or liquid meals. They may be curious about trying these products but don't get around to it until the event day. Big mistake! In some instances they discover (much to their dismay) that the unfamiliar food or drink gives them an upset stomach, heartburn, diarrhea, or cramps, an unpleasant situation that can affect performance and morale. As one woman lamented during a racing clinic (where free samples were readily available), "This sports drink has left a terrible taste in my mouth. Does anyone have any plain water I can have?" Good thing it was only a clinic!

Realize that there will be some occasions when the tried-and-true foods that you tolerate during training may not be tolerable during a race or special ride. Chalk that up to nervousness, not the food itself.

● **TOLERATING RIDE FOOD**—Enjoying a comfortable riding experience and a good workout depends on your ability to tolerate food before and during your ride. Gastrointestinal (GI) problems are not uncommon in cycling and run the gamut from nagging heartburn and fullness to vomiting and diarrhea. Such adverse reactions occur in an estimated 30 to 50 percent of endurance athletes. If you are prone to GI or other food-related problems while riding, the following information can help you develop a sports nutrition plan that works best for you.

Some of the factors that can affect the ability to tolerate ride food include:

- *The intensity of exercise.* The harder you work, the more likely you are to experience GI upset. You may be able to eat within ten minutes of an easy ride, an hour before a harder ride, but need to wait three hours before a sprint or hill workout. If you exercise at a pace that you can comfortably sustain for more than 30 minutes, you can likely both exercise and digest food at the same time. At this training pace, the blood flow to your stomach is 60 to 70 percent of normal and is adequate to maintain normal digestion processes. During high-intensity riding, as sprinting, racing, or hill climbing, your stomach gets about 20 percent of its normal blood flow. This slows digestion so that pre-exercise food will simply sit heavily during the ride, increasing your risk for GI problems.
- *The type of exercise.* Exercise that jostles the stomach, such as running, mountain biking, or cross racing, tends to cause more stomach upset than exercise where the body bounces less, such as road cycling. Practice eating during training for the type of event you plan to do.
- *The time of exercise.* Riding at a time you are not used to riding can affect your ability to comfortably tolerate food before exercising. Your stomach may tolerate lunchtime foods

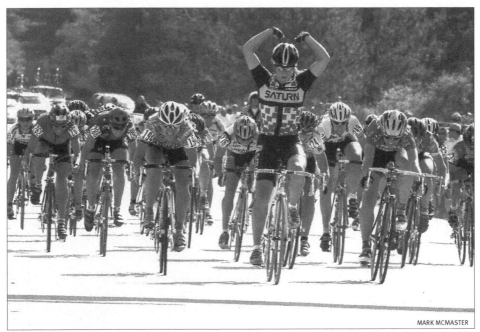

If you can't tolerate eating before an intense ride, plan to consume sports drinks during the ride. Experiment during training to know which brands—in which amounts—you can tolerate.

before your usual afternoon ride but not breakfast foods before an unusual morning ride. If you will participate in an event that will occur at an unfamiliar time, make sure you practice riding and eating at this time during training.

- *How nervous you are.* Nothing settles well when your stomach is in knots. Fuel-up sufficiently the day and night before if you know you will have a case of the jitters on event day.
- *Training status.* Cyclists who are new to the sport have more GI complaints than well-trained veterans whose bodies have adapted to their riding programs. Also, experienced riders have learned what works for them from many years of riding and have their nutrition regimen fine-tuned. If you are a novice rider, gradually increase your training volume and intensity so your body can adapt, and learn what you can and cannot handle.
- *Level of hydration.* Dehydration increases the risk of GI problems, so make sure you are well-hydrated before getting on the bike. Learn through training rides which beverages you can and cannot tolerate.

- *Volume of food eaten.* Large meals take longer to empty from the stomach and will leave you feeling like you are carrying a sack of bricks in your belly during the ride. The general rule of thumb for pre-ride food is to allow:
  - 3 to 4 hours for a large meal to digest
  - 2 to 3 hours for a smaller meal
  - 1 to 2 hours for a blended or liquid meal
  - Less than an hour for a small snack, as tolerated

  If you want to eat a full meal before an event but fear it will upset your stomach, simply allow ample time for it to digest by eating earlier. For example, if you'll be riding at 9 a.m., plan to eat your big breakfast by 6 a.m. If you'll ride at 7 a.m. you may need to get up at 4 a.m. to eat, and then go back to bed. For guidelines on eating during your ride, see chapter 11.

- *Composition of ride food.* Carbohydrates digest more quickly than fatty foods. Low-fat meals (such as those listed in *High-Carbohydrate Meal Suggestions*, page 101) digest easily and settle well. In comparison, high-fat meals such as bacon-and-egg breakfasts, cheeseburgers, tuna subs loaded with mayonnaise, and thick peanut butter sandwiches take longer to digest, linger in the stomach, and can contribute to a weighed-down feeling, if not nausea.

  A little fat, however, is appropriate. A slice of cheese on toast, some peanut butter on a bagel, or the fat in some brands of energy bars can provide both sustained energy and satiety during long rides. Note that some cyclists can break all the sports nutrition rules and do well with even very high-fat foods. After all, steak and eggs was the Olympic breakfast of champions for many years!

- *Consistency of the food.* Liquid foods leave the stomach faster than solid foods. If a bagel before your ride or a turkey sandwich during your ride upsets your stomach, then experiment with liquids, such as juice, a smoothie, or a canned liquid meal.

● **PRE-RIDE SUGAR**—Sugary carbohydrates, such as soft drinks, extra maple syrup, jellybeans, or sweetened juices, consumed 15 to 45 minutes before riding may cause hypoglycemia in sensitive individuals, leaving them fatigued, lightheaded, and

● HIGH-CARBOHYDRATE MEAL SUGGESTIONS

Some carbohydrate-based meal suggestions include tried-and-true favorites such as:

Breakfast: cold cereals, oatmeal and other hot cereals, multi-grain bagels, English muffins, pancakes, whole-wheat toast with jam, fruit, juice

Lunch: sandwiches (with wholesome bread being the "meat" of the sandwich), hearty broth-based or bean soups, thick-crust veggie pizza, low-fat fruit yogurt, low-fat milk, fruit, juice

Dinner: pasta, potato, or rice entrées, bean-and-rice burritos, bean, lentil, or pea soups, vegetables (especially corn, peas, winter squash, and sweet potato), baked beans, whole-grain breads and rolls, juice, fresh fruit

Snacks: low-fat flavored yogurt, pretzels, crackers, fig bars, frozen yogurt, dry cereal, leftover pasta, zwieback, whole-wheat toast, biscuit-type cookies, graham crackers, animal crackers, juice, low-fat milk, and canned, fresh, or dried fruits

shaky. If you think you may be sensitive to sugar, don't eat it! This includes sports drinks and gels. (Note that sugar taken during exercise generally does not contribute to a hypoglycemic reaction because muscles quickly use the sugar without the need for extra insulin.)

The best advice is for you to avoid the need for pre-ride sugary treats in the first place by eating appropriately-timed, nourishing meals prior to exercise. If you crave sugar before an afternoon training ride, you should have eaten a bigger breakfast and lunch. Skimping on meals may leave you looking for a last-minute sugary energizer that will not compensate for the lack of fuel earlier in the day.

● SUMMARY—

- Consume 800-1200 calories of a carbohydrate-rich meal 3 to 4 hours prior to riding to maximize your performance. Enjoy 100-300 calories of carbohydrate-rich food as tolerated before riding to top-off your glycogen stores and enhance your stamina and energy.

- Pre-ride carbohydrates help preserve muscle glycogen and reduce your risk of "hitting the wall." They also help prevent hypoglycemia, or "bonking," so you have the mental drive to finish the ride.
- In addition to offering physiological benefits, tried-and-true, pre-ride foods and beverages offer a psychological value: You don't waste energy worrying about what you ate (or didn't eat).
- Factors that affect your ability to tolerate pre-ride food include how hard you plan to ride, the time of day, your stress level, how hydrated you are, and kinds and amount of foods and drinks you consume.
- Always experiment during training to determine what pre-exercise menu works best for you to give you the most enjoyment and the best performance.

Words of wisdom from other cyclists... ━━━━━━━━━━━━━━━━━━

"For a training ride less than 1 to 2 hours, eating a good balanced breakfast pre-ride is preferable to consuming high-sugar sports foods while riding."
Khai Harbut, Plano, TX

"Initially, I couldn't eat before exercise or else I would get nauseated. Realizing I needed energy before heading out, I finally discovered that a glass of milk kick-starts me without ill effects."
Kim Holland, Maitland, FL

"For brevets that start at 3 or 4 a.m., I wake up an hour before start time, have a small amount of easy-to-digest protein (lemon yogurt works well for me), a bagel, and plenty of sports drink."
John McClellan, Groton, MA

"While my pre-ride breakfast is digesting, I stretch and drink from a liter of water. When I start to urinate, I know I'm hydrated."
Steve Chabra, New York, NY

CHAPTER 11

Foods and Fluids During Long Rides

BECOMING FATIGUED IS A MAJOR CONCERN OF MOST CYCLISTS, PARticularly long-distance cyclists. If you have ever "hit the wall" or "bonked," then you know how mental and physical exhaustion can slow you down, keep you from enjoying your ride, and at worst, leave you on the side of the road, waiting for the sag wagon.

You can prevent or delay the onset of fatigue during long rides by:
- preventing dehydration and
- preventing hypoglycemia (low blood sugar).

● **PREVENTING DEHYDRATION**—Sweat accounts for the majority of water lost from your body during exercise. Sweating is your body's way of dissipating heat to maintain a normal body temperature. In order to prevent dehydration during exercise you must replace sweat losses by drinking plenty of fluids.

Unfortunately by the time you may feel like drinking (i.e. your thirst kicks in), you are already dehydrated and probably have lost one percent or more of your body weight in sweat. As dehydration progresses, your breathing and heart rate increase, your ability to prevent overheating decreases, and fatigue sets in. Once dehydrated during exercise, you will have a very hard time correcting the imbalance.

Since your body's thirst mechanism is not a reliable signal to drink, plan to drink on a schedule before you feel thirsty. As a general rule, drink 8 ounces (240 milliliters), roughly 8 gulps,

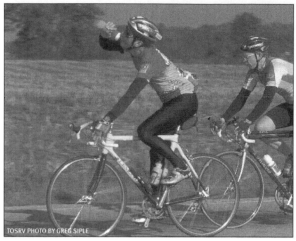
TOSRV PHOTO BY GREG SIPLE

Knowing your sweat rate helps you know how much to drink during your rides. Consume at least 16 ounces (480 milliliters) of fluid for every pound (.45 kilograms) of sweat you lose.

of water or sports drink every 15 to 20 minutes during hot and sweaty exercise. This is far less than what most cyclists would voluntarily consume.

To be safe, know your sweat rate and fluid targets (see chapter 8) and practice meeting your fluid goals during training. If you are not used to consuming this much fluid while biking, you can train your gut to handle this volume by gradually increasing your fluid intake during training rides. Marking your water bottles in 8-ounce (240-milliliter) increments or setting your watch or bike computer to remind you to drink at regular intervals can be helpful.

Do not drink more water than you can handle. The immediate solution to "stomach sloshing" is to stop drinking for a while. The long-term solution is to practice drinking during training, so your body can adapt to the appropriate fluid intake.

Here are a few tips on how to prevent dehydration.

- *Take advantage of every opportunity to drink.* Drink from and then top-off your water bottles (but do not over-hydrate) at every checkpoint, rest stop, or convenience store along the route.
- *Bring enough of your own preferred fluids for competitive or organized events.* Don't rely on the venue to provide water or your favorite sports drink. While riding drink frequently, and don't get so caught up in the excitement that you forget to drink and fall short of your fluid goals.
- *Plan water stops or bring a ride's supply.* For unsupported rides, select a route that includes water fountains, convenience stores, or cafes. If you are riding in a remote location, carry all the fluids that you need for the ride. Some cyclists use a portable hydration system that straps to the back. This offers the advantage of high volume: Large ones hold 3 quarts (~3 liters) or

more, enough for several hours of cycling. If you prefer water bottles, you can mount multiple bottle cages on your bike (on the frame, saddle, and handlebars) or carry extra filled bottles in jersey pockets or a pannier.

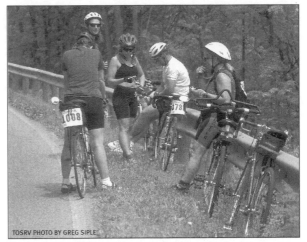

TOSRV PHOTO BY GREG SIPLE

If you plan to eat energy bars, gels, or regular food during your ride, also plan to drink plenty of water.

• *Become proficient at drinking while riding.* Practice your bike-handling skills every time you ride: drinking while pedaling, climbing, braking, or riding in a pack; drinking with either hand; switching water bottles from front cage to back; and retrieving bottles out of jersey pockets. The more comfortable you feel doing these things, the more likely you are to drink as frequently as you should, and the safer you are on the bike doing so.

For more information on fluids, water, and hydration, see chapter 8.

• **PREVENTING HYPOGLYCEMIA**—Because your brain controls your muscles and your ability to concentrate on the task at hand, you will ride well if your brain is well fed. The brain relies on glucose (blood sugar) for fuel. This glucose is derived from the carbohydrates that you consume and from carbohydrates (glycogen) stored in your liver. Hypoglycemia occurs when your blood sugar levels begin to fall. Referred to as "bonking," hypoglycemia makes you feel lightheaded, dizzy, irritable, and very tired. You may question if you can continue to ride. Judgment, decision-making, and alertness become impaired. These factors not only hurt performance and ruin a good ride, they put you at risk for accidents on the road.

You need to consume carbohydrates during your ride to prevent hypoglycemia and significantly improve your stamina. This is especially true if you have not fueled-up properly with

● POPULAR FOODS & FLUIDS DURING LONG RIDES

Depending on your body size and ability to tolerate food, target at least 200 to 300 calories of carbohydrates and 24 to 32 ounces (750 ml to 1000 ml) of fluid per hour while on the bike. Here is a listing of some popular foods and fluids—a list generated in part by the contributions and advice of many cyclists all over the world.

Foods	Amount	Calories	Carb. (g)	Protein (g)	Fat (g)
Almonds/peanuts	¼ cup	160	7	4	15
Bagel, plain	4-inch (89 g)	250	47	9	1
Banana	1 medium	105	26	1	0
Cheese, reduced-fat	1 oz.	80	0	7	6
Dates, dried	5	120	30	0	0
Fig Newtons	1	60	11	1	1
Go-Gurt (yogurt in a tube)	2.25 oz.	80	13	2	2
Granola bar, plain, hard	1 bar (28 g)	130	18	3	5
Kelloggs PopTart (blueberry frosted)	1	210	37	2	6
Oatmeal cookie	2½-inch cookie (28 g)	65	10	1	2
Orange	1 medium	70	17	1	0
Peanut butter and jelly sandwich	1 small	360	45	14	16
York Peppermint Patty	1.5 oz. patty	165	35	1	3
Raisins	⅓ cup	160	40	2	0
Snickers candy bar	2.16-oz. bar	280	37	6	14

Nutrition information from food labels and J. Pennington, 2004, Bowes & Church's Food Values of Portions Commonly Used, 18th ed. (Philadelphia: Lippincott, Williams & Wilkins).

a pre-ride meal, are dieting to lose weight, or ride first thing in the morning after an all-night fast. The amount of carbohydrate in a typical sports drink is adequate for shorter rides lasting 90 minutes or less.

For longer rides, the American College of Sports Medicine suggests about 50 grams of carbohydrate (or 200 calories) for a 150-pound (70-kg) cyclist each hour. More specifically, that's 0.3 grams carbohydrate per pound of body weight (or 0.7 g per kg) per hour while riding (ACSM 2009). More recent research (Juekendrup 2010) suggests cyclists can utilize 60 to 90 grams (240 to 360 calories) per hour of carbohydrates from a variety of sources, such as sports drinks, bananas, bagels, etc. Fueling with just one source of sugar can limit the absorption of that sugar.

For best results, consume some of your target carbohydrates

	Amount	Calories	Carb. (g)	Protein (g)	Fat (g)
Beverages					
Carnation Instant Breakfast	1.25-oz. packet	130	25	6	0
Cranberry juice cocktail	8 oz.	145	36	0	0
Defizzed cola	12 oz.	160	40	0	0
Chocolate low-fat milk	8 oz.	155	26	8	2
Orange juice	8 oz.	110	26	2	0
Energy Bars/Gels					
Clif	1 bar	240	45	10	4.5
Extran Endurance Bar	1 bar	225	50	1	2
Luna	1 bar	180	27	10	4
PowerBar Harvest	1 bar	240	45	7	4.5
PowerBar Performance	1 bar	230	45	10	2.5
SmartFuel WARPbar	1 bar	180	31	8	3.5
Gu	1 pack (32 g)	100	25	0	0
Hammer Gel	2 tbsp. (36 g)	90	23	0	0
Powdered Sports Drinks/Per 25 to 30 grams (2 Tablespoons)					
Accelerade	¾ scoop (27 g)	90	16	4	1
Cytomax	1 scoop (25 g)	95	20	0	0
Extran Thirst Quencher	1 scoop (28 g)	30	7	0	0
Gatorade	1½ scoop (30 g)	120	30	0	0
Hammer Perpetuem	¾ scoop (26 g)	98	20	2	1
Hammer Sustained Energy	1 scoop (28 g)	110	24	3	0
SmartFuel WarpAide	¾ scoop (30 g)	110	27	0	0

1 cup = 240 milliliters; 1 tablespoon = 15 milliliters; 1 ounce = 28 grams

every 15 to 20 minutes throughout the duration of the ride, rather than waiting until you are hungry (and you are already depleted) or loading-up once every couple of hours. Begin this process as soon as you get on the bike: Fuel early and often!

Practice consuming a variety of solid or liquid carbohydrates—juice, gels, fruit, granola bars, whatever—to see what works for you. Very fast riders and elite racers tend to prefer sports drinks or gels. And even if they cannot swallow a drink, just swishing a sports drink can enhance performance! (Beelen 2009)

Slower riders who don't hammer through their ride can thrive with a variety of regular foods and fluids. Despite popular belief, refined sugar (like jellybeans, sugar cubes, and soft drinks) can be a positive snack while cycling. During rides, we're talking "survival" and not "perfect nutrition"!

Some cyclists think they should train "on empty," without having eaten, believing they will burn more fat, hence lose more body fat, while riding. While it's true you might burn more fat, whether or not you will lose body fat depends on your calorie balance at the end of the day. That is, you can burn off 500 calories on a pre-breakfast ride, feel exhausted and starving afterwards, and then eat 1,000 calories of pancakes. No fat loss there!

Another reason competitive cyclists ride on empty is to train the body to burn more fat, so they can spare their limited muscle glycogen stores. As we said in chapter 10, this concept of "training low, competing high" needs more research to determine if this results in better performance and race results, or just mental toughness.

During training, devise a program for eating and drinking for riding so you know what, when, and how much you like to consume for the best performance. See *Popular Foods & Fluids During Long Rides* on pages 106-107 to help you devise your nutrition plan for riding.

Here are a few tips to help you prevent hypoglycemia:

- *Bring carbohydrates with you.* A jersey or jacket with multiple, easy-to-reach pockets is a good way to carry your snacks. You can grab the food while riding and avoid the need to stop to eat. If you prefer liquid carbohydrate, bring enough sports drink or other liquid for the ride. For longer distances, bring powered sports drinks to which you simply add water.
- *Know what foods and fluids you tolerate.* To avoid unwanted surprises such as heartburn, diarrhea, or upset stomach during an event, avoid foods or sports drinks that you have not tried during training. Your training rides are the time to sample unfamiliar food and drink.
- *Replenish your supplies along the way.* For long events ask friends to bring your requested fuel/fluid and meet you at designated areas along the course. Or else, plan a route that has stores where you can buy food and beverages.
- *Make a plan.* For stressful events, think ahead and make a clear plan before the event day. Plan what, when, and how you will eat and drink, and make sure you have practiced this in

training. This is especially important for less seasoned riders and those doing their first event. And be flexible—who knows what you will tolerate when your body and mind are pushed to the limit! Even tried-and-true favorites can become unpalatable.

- *Choose either solid or liquid carbohydrates.* Many cyclists prefer to drink their carbohydrates in the form of sugary fluid such as sports drink, diluted juice, or defizzed cola. Solid foods can work well, too, if you drink plenty of water and can tolerate the food.

- *Become proficient at eating while riding.* Practice your bike-handling/eating skills every time you ride. Practice getting food out of your jersey pocket, unwrapping it, and eating it while pedaling, coasting, or riding in a pack. If you are right-handed, keep food in the left pocket and reach back with the left hand so that your strongest hand/arm stays connected to the handlebar (do the opposite if you are left-handed). The more comfortable you are eating on the bike, the safer you'll be and the more likely you are to eat as much as you should.

- *Prepare and stash your bike food for easy access.* During training discover which foods are best to carry, open, and eat while riding. Before the ride, unwrap or tear open energy bars so there's no fussing with wrappers while riding. Portion your hourly food into separate small bags (and consume contents of one bag per hour). Figure out what to stash in which jersey pocket and what to tuck away in your bike bag. Some cyclists tape gel packets or energy bars to their handlebars or store unwrapped food directly in (clean) jersey pockets! Remember where you put your food and pack it the same way each time so that eating becomes a habit.

- *To save room and weight, carry powdered beverages or sports drinks.* This only applies if you will have access to water to reconstitute them.

- **SPORTS FOODS AND DRINKS**—As we have mentioned before, there is no magic to the special sports bars, gels, or drinks marketed to cyclists. These engineered products offer no nutritional advantage over regular food or drink. They do offer convenience in a pre-wrapped, easy, and portable package.

Whichever way you choose to consume your fuel is fine as long as it works for you.

Some cyclists find they tolerate commercial sports drinks better than other carbohydrate fluids such as juice or soft drinks. Sports drinks are dilute solutions of carbohydrates with a few electrolytes added to aid in absorption. They contain much less carbohydrate per ounce than juices and soft drinks (and solid foods).

You can dilute ordinary beverages with water (such as a 1:1 ratio of orange juice and water), add a dash of salt, and create a carbohydrate drink with a profile similar to a commercial sports drink (see the recipe on page 88).

Beware that while they may be fortified, commercial sports foods and drinks lack the vitamins and minerals, antioxidants, fiber, and other nutrients that natural foods contain. They also tend to be more expensive. The bottom line is choose a carbohydrate food or drink that you like and know you tolerate.

● **FOOD TOLERANCE**—Fear of stomach upset can deter some riders from eating during rides. On the other hand, fear of bonking can lead others to overeat during rides, leading to stomach upset. Experiment in training to find what works for you. Refer back to the previous chapter to *Tolerating Ride Food* on page 98 for tips about food before and during exercise.

Endurance cyclists, touring cyclists, and randonneurs who are on the bike for long hours and often days at a stretch can suffer from taste fatigue, especially if they are using only commercial sports foods. Sweet, high-carbohydrate foods and fluids all day long can become monotonous. Try a variety of standard foods and fluids during training, like sandwiches, bagels with peanut butter, and pretzels, to see what you tolerate. This way, if you begin to crave a hamburger in your 80th mile (or 8th hour or 8th day) you will know whether you can (or cannot) handle one.

● **FAT DURING EXERCISE**—While carbohydrates are an important fuel during exercise, eating a little fat is okay, too. Fat-containing foods provide sustained energy. A little fat—such as that in peanut butter, cheese, chocolate, granola bar, or cookie—helps food digest more slowly and therefore can provide longer lasting energy for people who will be riding for more than a couple hours.

● **PROTEIN DURING EXERCISE**—During endurance exercise, your body breaks down a little of its muscle protein. Consuming some protein before, during, and after exercise can help to offset this loss and improve protein balance (Koopman et al. 2004). Some popular protein foods include an egg or milk with the pre-ride breakfast, chocolate milk or nuts during the ride, and turkey (in a sandwich) after the ride. Many sports drinks and bars are fortified with protein. Of course, protein should never up-stage carbohydrates as your primary fuel for cycling.

● **SUMMARY**—All too often riders hold off until after their ride to enjoy a good meal. They end up needlessly fatigued and overly hungry. Why wait until after your ride to enjoy the fuel that could have enhanced your performance and enjoyment during the ride?

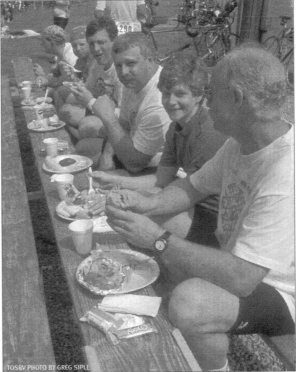

- The fluids and foods that you consume during your rides should be an extension of your carbohydrate-rich daily training diet.
- Preventing dehydration and low blood sugar (hypoglycemia) are the keys to preventing fatigue.
- To prevent dehydration, know your sweat rate and replace fluids accordingly. Drink on a schedule, targeting 8 ounces (240 milliliters) of fluid more or less, depending on your sweat rate, every 15 to 20 minutes.
- To prevent hypoglycemia, target at least 0.3 grams

TOSRV PHOTO BY GREG SIPLE

While eating during your biking events, eat wisely so the food doesn't talk back to you when you get back on the bike.

carbohydrates per pound of body weight (0.7 g per kg) during each hour of riding; that's 40-60 grams of carbohydrate (150-250 calories) per hour. Many riders can tolerate and ride better with even more carbs (60-90 g per hour). Consume carbohydrates every 15-20 minutes throughout the ride.

- Sports foods, gels, and drinks while easy and convenient, are costly and offer no better nutrition than standard foods. They lack many of the nutrients that real food provides.
- Learn through trial and error during training what foods and fluids settle best and contribute to top performance.
- During training: develop a feeding and fluid plan for the event; learn your fluid and calorie targets and which foods and fluids you need to achieve these targets; and know how you will access your foods and fluids during your event.

Words of wisdom from other cyclists... ▬▬▬▬▬▬▬▬▬▬▬▬

"I started riding to lose weight. I thought I would lose more weight on my first century ride if I didn't eat much, so I brought only one PowerBar, two gels, and no money for food. Sixty miles into the ride, I was toast. I made it back, but it was pretty ugly and I was wiped out for three days after that ride."
Lindsay Langford, Indianapolis, IN

"Eat even when you're tired, not hungry, you hate your food choices, or it seems like you just ate. Try to keep a regular schedule and check it on your watch. This is not about things tasting good or feeling hungry; this is about having gas in the tank."
Elmar Stefke, Berkeley, CA

"For longer rides, it's always a good idea to hydrate and fuel early and consistently to keep your energy up. I like to have most all of my necessary calories per hour in each 20- to 24-ounce bottle. That way, I don't have to fumble with anything in my pockets if the pace picks up. If there is time for a stop, my favorites are a few dates or Rice Krispies Treats because they are very palatable and easy to digest."
Kristen Christiansen, Henderson, NV

"Always bring some food with you no matter what. I have bonked many times on 'one- hour rides' that got extended due to mechanical problems that caused mayhem."
Sarah Lanphier

"I match eating with intensity. If things are going to be low-key for a while, that sandwich is okay. If I don't know, a gel will do. If I'm going to push it to the limit (a hill or sprint) anytime soon, I'll get my carbs from a bottle of sports drink."
Elmar Stefke, Berkeley, CA

"During very long rides, I found that I couldn't continue to eat the same energy bars or drinks so had to change-up often. In the end, eating real food was always the best. Regular food seems to sit better and is more satisfying."
Marcia Gibbs, California

"In hard races it can be difficult to take in fuel and hydrate properly. If you are really maxed out, you may feel like reaching for a gel packet but can't find a point to do this comfortably. I try to know the course and plan for those easier points to reach for the gel. Sometimes, I watch to see when the top guys are fueling and do the same."
Jerry Jacobs, Wayland, MA

"For long rides (6+ hours), I love dried mango. It has the exact amount of sugar to make you feel better. It tastes great, doesn't spoil, and you can eat it while you are riding. Weather doesn't affect it, and it doesn't dry your mouth."
Marco Otilio Pena Diaz, McAllen, TX

"Due to the hazard of crashing, I actually stop my bike, find a shady spot with seating, and eat an unhurried snack. This seems like the sensible and enjoyable thing to do."
John Klever, Denver, CO

"During a century, I had a hefty peanut butter sandwich and lots of water at one of the 25-mile rest stops. It was just what I needed, or so I thought. A half-mile into the long hill that followed I began to feel queasy, and it all came up. Now, I won't eat more than a couple of handfuls at a time, but I eat often. At rest stops, I eat half of what they give me and put the rest in my pocket for later."
Rich Lesnik, San Francisco, CA

"During a double century, the taste of food changes over the course of time. The sweet stuff that tasted great at the beginning is repulsive later on, when tart and salty foods start tasting much better."
Elmar Stefke, Berkeley, CA

CHAPTER 12

Recovery: What to Eat After Hard Rides

JUST AS FUELING BEFORE AND DURING A LONG, HARD RIDE IS IMPORTANT, so is refueling afterwards. Your post-ride sports diet is critical for a full and speedy recovery. By replenishing depleted glycogen stores, rehydrating body tissues, restoring electrolytes, and providing your muscles with the nutrients they need to heal damaged tissue, you'll be able to endure repeated days (and weeks) of hard training, racing, or touring. Poor recovery practices take their toll, limiting how hard you can train, how fast you can improve, how good you feel on and off the bike and ultimately, how much you enjoy the overall biking experience.

Note: If you are a recreational cyclist who does not exhaust yourself during your 30- to 60-minute pleasure-ride, you need not worry about your recovery diet. You have not depleted yourself and so you have small losses that will be easily replaced via standard meals.

● **RECOVERY FLUIDS**—Your first priority after a hard ride is to replace fluid losses as soon as possible. Ideally, you have minimized a fluid deficit by drinking plenty of fluids while riding and replacing sweat losses as they occurred (see chapter 8). Recovery is quick when you've prevented dehydration!

Here are answers to some of the questions you may have about rehydration:

When and how much should I drink after a hard ride?—As soon as you get off the bike, drink enough to quench your

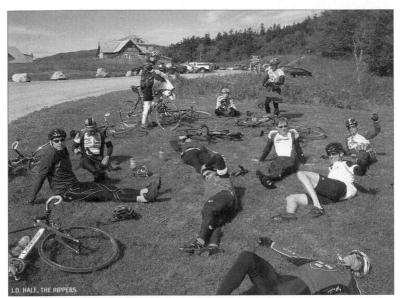

Recovery is much easier if you take time to eat and drink appropriately during the ride.

thirst, and then drink more. You might not feel thirsty immediately or for several hours, but your body may still need fluid. Your goal is to have a significant quantity of pale-colored urine.

Make sure recovery fluids will be available at the end of your ride, wherever that will be. Plan to end your ride at a home or a convenience store, or pack your favorite recovery fluids with you in an ice-filled cooler to take along in the car. It is also a good idea to keep a gallon of water in your car so you will have fluid available when you or your thirsty companions need it.

What's best to drink for recovery? Are sports drinks preferable?—Good fluid choices include any that taste good to you so you'll drink plenty of them: water, juices, chocolate milk, fruit smoothies, sports drinks, soft drinks, lemonade, sweetened ice tea, or whatever you prefer. Here is information on some popular fluids to help you choose what is best for you:

• *Water.* Plain water provides fluid but not the carbohydrates you need to replenish depleted muscle glycogen. Thus, you should eat carbohydrate-rich foods with the water, such as a bagel, fruit, or energy bar. Because sodium enhances fluid absorption and retention, enjoy some salty foods with your water, such as pretzels or salted nuts, especially if you were

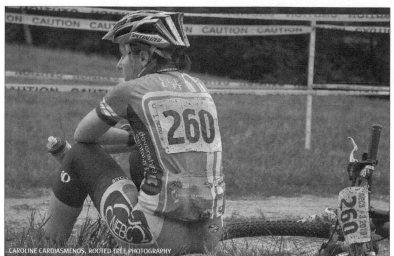

Begin consuming recovery foods and fluids as soon as you get off the bike to rapidly refuel depleted muscles.

biking in hot weather and have lost a lot of sweat. Brothy soup is often welcomed after chilly rides.

- *Soft drinks.* Although they lack nutritional value and are filled with empty calories, soft drinks offer both carbohydrates and fluids. Cola offers caffeine, which for some may provide welcome stimulation. Historically, athletes have been told to avoid caffeine, believed to be a diuretic that would hamper efforts to replace fluids. But now we know that caffeine has no diuretic effect in athletes who are accustomed to consuming it and is not likely to hurt recovery (Armstrong 2002). Because soft drinks lack sodium, you should also consume some crackers, baked chips, or other salty foods.

- *Juices.* Fruit and vegetable juices are excellent choices because they are carbohydrate-rich and they offer the vitamin C your body needs to optimize healing. Salty vegetable juices, such as V8 or tomato juice, aid in fluid absorption and retention. Fruit juice, like water and soft drinks, lacks sodium, so consume a muffin, sandwich, or other salt-containing foods with your fruit juice.

- *Sports drinks.* Commercial fluid replacers (such as Gatorade) are designed to be taken during exercise. They are dilute solutions of sugar in water with a small amount of sodium added. After exercise, you will get many more carbohydrates

THE CYCLIST'S FOOD GUIDE: FUELING FOR THE DISTANCE

per ounce by drinking juice. For example, you would have to drink 48 ounces (1.3 liters) of a sports drink to get the carbohydrates contained in just 16 ounces (480 milliliters) of cranberry-apple juice.

- *Chocolate milk.* Any flavored low-fat milk or soymilk—chocolate, vanilla, strawberry—is an excellent recovery food because it offers all that your body wants: water to replace sweat losses, carbs to refuel, protein to repair, and sodium to enhance fluid retention. Stock your cooler or refrigerator with this tasty treat!
- *Commercial recovery drinks.* Commercial drinks (such as Muscle Milk) contain many of the same nutrients you get in chocolate milk, but at a higher price. They are not "better," just more expensive.

Is beer a good recovery fluid?—Beer is often a part of post-ride festivities. But when you are dehydrated and hungry, drinking alcohol on an empty stomach can hit you like a ton of bricks. Similarly, wine and other alcoholic beverages lack the carbohydrates you need to replenish your glycogen stores. A 12-ounce bottle of beer has just 11 to 13 grams of carbohydrates, fewer carbs than a slice of bread.

Drinking alcohol post-ride impairs glycogen synthesis by displacing carbohydrates from your recovery diet (Burke et al. 2003). That is, if you are drinking beer, you are not drinking orange juice or chocolate milk! If you plan to consume alcohol post-ride, first drink plenty of non-alcoholic fluids and eat some salty, high-carbohydrate foods. Then, enjoy a beer or two in moderation.

For more on recovery fluids, see *Comparing Fluid Replacers* in chapter 8.

- **RECOVERY CARBOHYDRATES**—The second priority after exhaustive riding is to replenish depleted glycogen (carbohydrate) stores. Eat carbohydrate-rich foods as soon as tolerable after a hard ride and continue for several hours. Cyclists who fail to recover with adequate carbohydrates will lack the fuel and energy needed to ride strongly the next day. This is a particular concern for long-distance touring cyclists, racers, and those who train hard every day (or twice a day).

In addition to recovery carbohydrates, you should eat a daily diet that is carbohydrate-based, with abundant grains and

● RECOMMENDED CARBOHYDRATE INTAKE FOR RECOVERY

Your muscles are most receptive to replacing depleted glycogen stores immediately after exercise. For optimal recovery, consume approximately 0.5 gram of carbohydrate per pound (1.0 gram per kilogram) of body weight each hour following exercise until your regular eating pattern can be resumed. You should also include a little protein (10-20 g) for muscle recovery.

Carbohydrates for recovery per hour after exercise:

Body weight	Carb. (g)	Body weight	Carb. (g)
120 lb (55 kg)	60	170 lb (77 kg)	85
130 lb (60 kg)	65	180 lb (82 kg)	90
140 lb (64 kg)	70	190 lb (86 kg)	95
150 lb (70 kg)	75	200 lb (90 kg)	100
160 lb (73 kg)	80	210 lb (95 kg)	105

cereals, starchy vegetables (peas, potatoes), fruits, and legumes (dried beans and peas, lentils, hummus). As a guideline, carbohydrate foods such as these should take up half to three-quarters of the space on your plate. This will help you to avoid the gradual and chronic glycogen depletion that can occur with repeated days and weeks of hard riding. Here are answers to some of the questions cyclists often ask about carbs.

When should I eat after my rides?—As soon as possible after hard exercise, you should begin replenishing your glycogen stores by consuming carbohydrates. We say as soon as possible because the most rapid glycogen synthesis occurs within 60 to 90 minutes following hard exercise. This is particularly important for riders who train hard on repeated days or who train more than once a day. Glycogen stores can be completely restored within 24 hours or sooner if the intake and timing of carbohydrate is right. If you need to rapidly refuel, we recommend starting the process of refueling within 15 minutes of getting off the bike.

How many carbohydrates do I need to recover?—For optimal glycogen recovery, you should consume about 0.5 gram of carbohydrate per pound (1.0 gram per kilogram) of body weight

Here is the carbohydrate and protein content of some selected recovery fluids and foods. Please refer to the table on pages 106-107 for more items.

Fluids	Amount	Calories	Carb. (g)	Protein (g)
Grapefruit juice	1 cup	95	22	0
V8 Juice	1 cup	50	10	0
Soymilk	1 cup	120	12	10
Lemonade	2 cups	150	35	0
Chocolate low-fat milk	1 cup	155	26	8
Foods				
Baked potato or sweet potato w/skin	1 large	280	60	7
Chicken-rice or lentil soup	1 cup	130	20	9
Baked beans	1 cup	235	50	15
Fruit yogurt (low-fat)	1 cup	225	40	8
Frozen yogurt (low-fat)	1 cup	230	35	6
Jelly, jam, honey, maple syrup, or sugar	1 tablespoon	50	13	0
Bagel	1 large	330	65	12
White or whole-wheat bread	1 slice	65-90	15-20	2-4
Cornflakes with 4 oz. milk	1 cup cereal	150	35	7
Oatmeal, cooked	1 cup	145	25	6
Rice, boiled	1 cup	265	55	5
Pretzels	10 twists	110	25	2
Peanut butter and jelly sandwich	1 sandwich	360	45	14
Hamburger (McDonald's)	1 small	280	35	13
Cheese pizza (Pizza Hut, 12-inch)	¼ pie	500	56	22
Bean burrito without cheese (Taco Bell)	1 small	300	55	10
Spaghetti with tomato sauce	1½ cups	230	45	9
Turkey sub (Subway)	6-inch	280	45	18
Commercial Recovery Drinks				
Endurox R4	2 scoops	270	52	13
Smartfuel BioFix	2 scoops	290	60	11
Cytomax Recovery	2 scoops	350	18	26
Hammer Recoverite	2 scoops	166	32	10

Nutrition information from food labels, product websites, USDA National Nutrient Database (online), and J. Pennington, 2004, Bowes & Church's Food Values of Portions Commonly Used, 18th ed. (Philadelphia: Lippincott, Williams & Wilkins)

1 cup = 240 milliliters; 1 tablespoon = 15 milliliters

The optimal refueling plan includes plenty of carbohydrates to restore glycogen, some protein to help heal damaged muscles, and sodium and potassium to replace that lost in sweat. If circumstances prevent you from sitting down to a recovery meal (or if you have no appetite) for several hours after your ride, you should consume enough carbohydrates immediately following your ride by drinking fluids and nibbling on snacks on a schedule. (To find out how many carbohydrates you need for recovery, see page 118.) And don't forget to drink plenty of water, too! Here are some healthful recovery choices that offer carbohydrate, protein, sodium, and potassium:

- Apple juice + Fig Newtons + salted almonds
- Yogurt + orange juice or fresh fruit + salted pretzels
- Chocolate milk + salted crackers
- Bagel + apple + cheese or peanut butter
- Hot or cold cereal + milk or soymilk + banana or raisins
- Pasta + tomato sauce + meat, seafood, chicken, or cheese
- Pancakes + blueberries + maple syrup
- Fruit + milk + fruit yogurt + a pinch of salt (in a smoothie)
- Vegetable, bean, or noodle soup + bread or crackers + milk
- Small hamburger, soy burger, or turkey sub + orange juice
- Peanut butter and jelly (or honey) sandwich + apple juice
- Baked potato + cheese + ketchup or salsa
- Thick-crust cheese or veggie-cheese pizza

each hour after getting off the bike until you are able to sit down to a regular meal. A 150-pound (70-kilogram) cyclist needs approximately 75 grams (300 calories) of carbohydrates per hour for several hours after exercise.

Note it's the amount of carbohydrate not the calories that is important for recovery. You should consume 75 grams (300 calories) of carbohydrates, not just 300 calories of anything (if you weigh 150 pounds or 70 kilograms). For example, an energy bar has close to 300 calories, but it may have far less than 75 grams of carbohydrates. In this case, you should eat two energy bars or drink enough orange juice with the bar to meet your carbohydrate goal. If you eat a 300-calorie sandwich (such a turkey or peanut butter sandwich), you likely are getting only 30 to 40 grams of carbohydrates, so be sure to also drink juice, put extra honey on the peanut butter, or snack on some dried fruit.

Most cyclists naturally get repeated doses of carbs without even thinking about it. They chug a chocolate milk after an early morning training ride, stretch, shower, then have a bowl of cereal, then a mid-morning bagel and juice, then a banana, and then lunch...

What are the best recovery carbohydrates?—Although all carbohydrates will help to replenish your depleted glycogen stores, easily digestible fruits, vegetables, and starches/grains should be the major carbohydrate choice in recovery meals. This is because the more easily the food is digested, the faster it is converted to glucose in the blood and the quicker your muscles have the substrate they need for making glycogen. Popular choices include banana, bagel, potato, breakfast cereal, orange juice, and honey, just to name a few.

If exercise kills your appetite or if even the thought of post-exercise food makes you nauseated, you can drink the carbohydrates (and simultaneously provide your body with the fluid it needs to recover). This is why ginger ale, fruit smoothies, and chicken noodle soup are popular choices for many cyclists. With time, your hunger will return. For some people, this may not be until the next day.

● **RECOVERY PROTEIN**—Eating a small amount of protein along with recovery fluids and carbohydrates can improve the body's protein balance, enhance muscle repair and reduce muscle soreness (Flakoll et al. 2004). If you are eating enough calories and carbohydrates, eating protein does not significantly improve the rate of muscle glycogen replacement (Jentjens et al. 2001, Zachweija 2002). Most cyclists consume more than enough protein on a daily basis. Refer to chapter 6 for more on protein.

Should I drink a protein shake after a hard ride?—No. If you fill up on protein, you will not fill up on carbohydrates. Similarly, don't fill up on the post-ride barbecued chicken and overlook the bread, potato, or pasta! The priority is refueling muscles with carbs.

While adequate protein is necessary to repair and rebuild muscles damaged by hard exercise, you do not need to eat a high-protein diet. Your recovery drink should have three or four times more carbs than protein. Add a big banana or juice to that protein shake, or more simply, choose chocolate milk!

What if I crave protein?—Many cyclists report craving protein, particularly red meat, after hard exercise. If that is the case for you, eat some (lean) steak and enjoy a large potato and rolls with it. This balance will help you rebuild and refuel, as well as enjoy the process.

● **RECOVERY ELECTROLYTES**—Electrolytes are electrically charged particles that help the body function normally. Some of the more familiar electrolytes include sodium, potassium, calcium, and magnesium. Calcium and magnesium help muscles contract and relax. Sodium and potassium help water stay in the right balance inside and outside of cells. Sodium is the electrolyte lost in the highest concentration in sweat, followed by potassium. Most cyclists will not deplete their body's electrolyte stores under ordinary circumstances in rides lasting under four hours. You lose proportionally more water than electrolytes during exercise, so your first need is to replace the fluid.

Here a few answers to common concerns about replacing electrolyte losses:

How much sodium and potassium do I lose in sweat?—
- One pound or 16 ounces (0.5 kilograms or 0.5 liter) of sweat contains on average 400 milligrams sodium and 100 milligrams potassium.
- Depending on your sweat rate, you might lose 1 to 4 pounds of sweat (0.5 to 2 kilograms) in each hour of sweaty exercise.
- In three hours of sweaty exercise, you may lose 1,200 to 4,500 milligrams of sodium (2 to 6 percent of your body stores) and 300 to 1,200 milligrams of potassium (0.001 to 0.007 percent of your stores). These losses are relatively insignificant and are easily restored by consuming regular foods and fluids during recovery and subsequent meals.

Do I need extra salt to recover what I lost in sweat?—
Probably not. You will easily replace the sodium lost in sweat

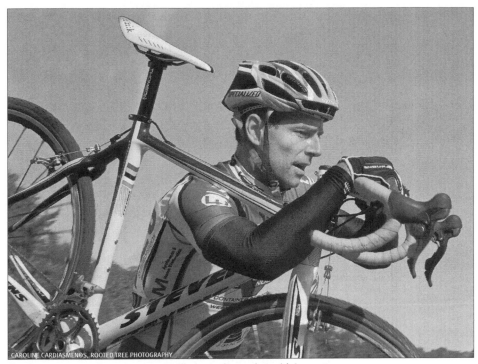

Good recovery practices assure you will always be ready to ride!

by enjoying ordinary foods. Sodium is found in foods naturally and is also a part of salt (1 teaspoon, or 5 grams, contains
2,300 milligrams of sodium). A recovery snack of chocolate
milk and a bagel with peanut butter contains about 1,000 milligrams of sodium.

Keep in mind that the longer and harder you exercise, the
hungrier you'll get and the more sodium-containing foods and
fluids you'll consume. You'll easily get more than enough sodium during and after your ride. Some cyclists say they crave
salt. If this is the case, simply listen to your body and enjoy
more salty foods.

Cyclists who need extra salt are those who ride in the heat
the entire day, tour in hot weather for multiple days, or train in
cold weather yet do their event (race, tour, etc.) in warm
weather. Ultra-distance riders, who ride day-and-night for multiple days, must pay particular attention to prevent sodium
depletion (hyponatremia) in all climates. To get extra salt, you
do not need salt tablets. Consuming salty and salted foods

gives you plenty of sodium: pasta with tomato sauce, pizza, turkey-and-cheese sub, V8 or tomato juice, salad dressings, pickles, olives, soup, salted nuts. Some ultra-distance riders simply lick a small packet of salt from their palm or suck on a bouillon cube. Tastes great if you crave it!

Note that commercial sports foods and fluids are often relatively poor sources of sodium (and potassium) compared with ordinary foods (see pages 78 and 87.) Check food labels and you may be surprised at the sodium content of many everyday foods.

Because recovery can start *before* you exercise, you can also consume salty foods, such as chicken broth or ramen noodles before extended sweaty exercise. This way, the sodium will be in your system, helping to retain fluid and maintain hydration. Experiment with consuming pre-exercise sodium during training.

Do I need extra potassium?—As with sodium, you lose some potassium when you sweat, but you are unlikely to deplete your body stores. Potassium in found in foods naturally, particularly in fruits, vegetables, and milk. You can easily replace potassium losses, for example, by eating a banana (450 milligrams potassium), nibbling on raisins (¼ cup = 300 milligrams potassium), or having a potato with dinner (800 milligrams potassium). On page 125 is a list of popular recovery foods and their potassium content. Some of these foods also work well during long rides (see chapter 11).

● **RECOVERY FOR CYCLISTS WHO WANT TO LOSE FAT**—If you are trying to shed undesired body fat, recovery is not the time to do it. In addition to needless fatigue, denying yourself adequate nourishment for recovery can lead to extreme hunger, carbohydrate cravings, and out-of-control food binges that contribute to weight gain.

Your best bet for reducing body fat is to refuel appropriately and then cut back on calories later in the evening. Your goal is to have energy during the day for cycling; you can then eat less at night and lose weight when you are sleeping, not training.

Ideally, you should try to shed extra body fat during the off-season or early-season training when you are not putting such

● POTASSIUM IN COMMONLY EATEN FOODS

During three hours of moderately sweaty riding, you might lose 300-1,200 milligrams of potassium. To replace this electrolyte you can include some of these popular high-potassium foods in your recovery plan. Also see *Comparing Fluid Replacers* on page 78.

Potassium: *Excellent sources include fruits, juices, vegetables, and dairy products.*

Food	Amount	Potassium (mg)
Potato, sweet or white, baked	1 large	715-845
Baked beans	1 cup	750
Cantaloupe	¼ melon	500
Orange juice	1 cup	475
V8 juice	1 cup	470
Banana	1 medium	450
Milk, chocolate low-fat	1 cup	425
Vegetable soup	1 cup	395
Milk, low-fat	1 cup	380
Fruit yogurt	1 cup	450
Raisins	¼ cup	300

Sports drinks and foods are generally poor sources of potassium:

	Amount	Potassium (mg)
Gatorade	8 oz.	30
Accelerade	8 oz.	40
Cytomax	8 oz.	80
Clif Bar	1 bar	210
PowerBar Recovery Bar	1 bar	85
GU Roctane	1 packet	55

1 cup = 240 milliliters; 1 ounce. = 30 milliliters

Nutrition information from food labels, USDA National Nutrient Database (online), and J. Pennington, 2004, Bowes & Church's Food Values of Portions Commonly Used, 18th ed. (Philadelphia: Lippincott, Williams & Wilkins)

physical demands on your body. For more on weight and reduction of body fat see chapter 16.

● **CELEBRATING AFTER A BIG EVENT**—A celebration is in order when you have completed the event for which you have been training long and hard. At the end of a race, randonnée, or tour, please relax, enjoy yourself, be proud of your accomplishment—

and, of course, munch on tasty carb-protein reward foods! If you have several days before the next event, you need not be obsessive with your recovery diet; you will not be demanding much from your muscles for a while. They need time to rest, heal, and refuel.

If you celebrate with beer, wine, or Champagne, be sure to at least eat some snacks first, so that you are not drinking alcohol on an empty stomach. Plan to first enjoy some juice or soft drink to supply your muscles with water and carbohydrates. A nice massage, a gentle swim, or very light ride to loosen stiff muscles are other helpful recovery ideas.

• SUMMARY—

- Refueling after hard rides is essential to replenish depleted glycogen and fluid stores, heal damaged muscles, and prepare your body for your next ride.
- Eat or drink carbohydrates within 15 minutes of getting off the bike, and then keep snacking on carbohydrates for the next few hours.
- Drink enough post-ride recovery fluids to quench your thirst, then drink more. Your goal is to have pale-colored urine in significant quantities.
- Eating a little protein with your recovery carbohydrates may enhance glycogen synthesis and muscle repair and reduce muscle soreness, but your focus should remain on carbohydrates and fluid.
- Consume potassium-rich fruits and juices, and salty foods and fluids to replace electrolyte losses. Commercial fluid replacement and recovery beverages are convenient, but standard foods and fluids can do the job just fine.
- Plan ahead so recovery foods and fluids will be available to you at the end of your ride or workout.
- Enjoy the refueling process...it's part of cycling's pleasures.

"Prepare a cooler for after the ride.
Pack it full of salty foods, such as pretzels, hummus,
ham sandwich with mustard, and cold chocolate milk."
Paula Mrowczynski-Hernandez, Houston, TX

"My favorite recovery drink is 12 ounces of chocolate milk
blenderized with one tablespoon of peanut butter and one banana."
Shaun Riebl, Deerield Beach, FL

"I drink a glass of juice or chocolate milk
(or whatever high-carb drink is in the fridge) within 10 minutes
of walking in the house from a hard or long ride.
I'll also grab something salty—a handful of salty baked chips,
sunflower seeds, or pretzel sticks—because I'm craving salt.
I've noticed a direct correlation: eat sooner, recover sooner...
feel better, ride better!"
Louise Wilcox, Reading, MA

CHAPTER 13

Event Week: Nutrition Preparations

I F YOU ARE PREPARING FOR A RACE, TRIATHLON, CENTURY, BREVET, OR any other endurance event that lasts for more than 90 minutes, you should saturate your muscles and liver with glycogen. These stored carbohydrates influence how long you can enjoy exercising. But carbo-loading requires more than just eating a pile of pasta the night before an event. What you do during the week leading up to your important ride can make or break your ability to successfully complete the distance you've been training for.

● **STORED CARBOHYDRATE AND GLYCOGEN**—In comparison to the approximately 1,800 to 2,000 calories stored as carbohydrates (glycogen), the average lean 150-pound (70-kilogram) man has 60,000 to 100,000 calories stored as fat, enough to ride several thousand miles! Unfortunately for cyclists and other endurance athletes, fat cannot be used exclusively for fuel because the muscles need carbohydrates to burn fat. Therefore, carbohydrates are a limiting factor for endurance athletes.

The amount of glycogen you use during cycling depends on how hard you ride and your level of training. Generally speaking, the greater the intensity of the ride, the more glycogen you use. Riding at high intensity, as in all-out sprinting, you burn primarily glycogen; at low intensity, you burn primarily fat. This explains why you may be able to ride casually for several hours, but not at a fast racing pace for more than an hour or two.

When your muscle glycogen stores run out, you feel exhausted and your physical strength quickly fades. When

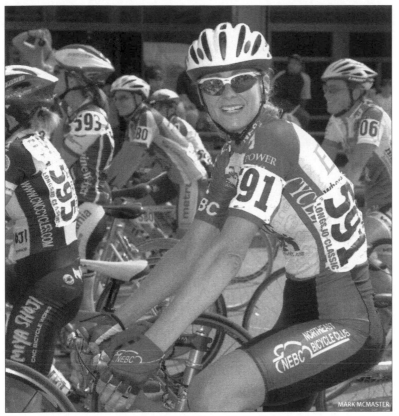

While waiting for your event to start, think positively. Trust that your body is well-fueled, well-trained, and ready to perform at its best.

your liver glycogen diminishes, you become hypoglycemic: Your blood sugar drops, you feel irritable, and your mental stamina rapidly declines. These conditions, known as "hitting the wall" and "bonking," are preventable if you saturate your body with carbohydrates before the ride and also replenish carbohydrates by eating and drinking during the ride. See chapters 10 and 11 for information on fueling before and during rides.

Your muscles' ability to store glycogen increases through training. Well-trained muscles can store 20 to 50 percent more glycogen than untrained muscles. With training, your muscles are also able to burn more fat. This change enhances endurance capacity and helps explain why elite riders can ride hard for hours without tiring.

• **YOUR DAILY TRAINING DIET**—Pre-event pasta meals have long been a carbo-loading tradition among cyclists. But for optimal glycogen storage, you should "carbo-load" not just the day before an event but also every day during your training. Cyclists who eat a carbohydrate-based diet can:

• Prevent chronic glycogen depletion.
• Train better because their muscles are better fueled, and then ride better on event day.
• Continue eating the same tried-and-true foods pre-event, so there are no unwanted surprises like stomach discomfort tor other problems. The last thing you want to do is change your diet before an event.

Your daily carb-based diet should be balanced with an appropriate amount of protein and fat (see chapters 6 and 7). Enjoy grain products, like bread, cereal, pasta, or rice, as the foundation of every meal and snack, along with plenty of fruits and vegetables and smaller amounts of protein foods and dairy products.

To help you avoid nutritional mistakes and reduce unwanted surprises on event day:

• *Practice eating your pre-event meals during training.* If your event will begin in the morning, practice eating breakfast; for afternoon events, breakfast and lunch. If you will travel to your race or ride, be sure your tried-and-true foods will be available for event day. You may need to bring all of your foods and drinks with you in a cooler.

• *Train at the time your event will occur.* If your race starts at noon, do some training rides at noon; if it begins at 6:00 a.m., include some early morning rides in your training. Learn how to eat and drink before, during, and after these times.

• *Learn how much pre-exercise food you can eat and then still ride comfortably.* This is particularly important for cyclists who ride at high intensity and have more difficulty digesting and tolerating pre-ride food. These may include racers or those on tour who face a hilly day.

• *Practice drinking the sports drinks and foods that will be available on the ride or at the event as well as any mid-ride foods you plan to eat.* This way, you will know what you can tolerate and what works best for you.

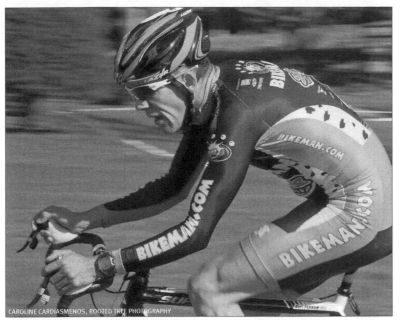

Carbo-load your muscles and liver with glycogen the days before your competitive event or endurance ride by tapering your training and eating your usual high-carbohydrate sports diet.

● **THE WEEK BEFORE THE EVENT**—The biggest change during the week before an event should be in your training, not in your eating. Taper your training so that your muscles have the opportunity to become fully saturated with glycogen. Do not engage in last-minute hard training that taps into glycogen stores and burns carbohydrates rather than allows them to be stored. With tapering, the 600 or more calories you would expend during a day's training can be stored as fuel in your muscles and liver.

Maintain your tried-and-true, high-carbohydrate training diet throughout your taper week. Drastic changes commonly lead to an upset stomach, diarrhea, or constipation. For example, carbo-loading on an unusually high amount of fruits and juices might cause diarrhea; too many white-flour, low-fiber bagels, breads, and pasta might lead to constipation.

If you are a competitive cyclist who races every weekend or multiple days in a row and have a training schedule that does not allow you to taper, you must be very diligent about maintaining a high-carbohydrate diet and consuming adequate carbohydrates during training and during your events.

These menus are appropriate for a 150-pound (70-kilogram) cyclist who needs about 4 grams carbohydrate per pound of body weight (8 grams per kilogram) to adequately carbo-load. The menus also supply an appropriate balance of protein and fats.

3,200 Total Calories	Calories	Carbs. (g)
Breakfast:	**840**	**172**
Wheaties, 2 cups	220	48
Milk, 1% low-fat, 8 oz.	100	12
Bagel, 1 (3.5 oz.)	300	55
Honey, 1 Tbsp	60	17
Orange juice, 12 oz.	160	40
Lunch:	**960**	**156**
Whole grain bread, 2 slices (2 oz.)	200	40
Peanut butter, 2 Tbsp	200	8
Jelly, 2 Tbsp	100	25
Fruit yogurt, 8 oz.	230	35
Pretzels, 2 oz.	230	48
Snack:	**240**	**52**
Apple, 1 large (7 oz.)	120	30
Graham crackers, 4 squares	120	22
Dinner:	**800**	**115**
Chicken breast, 5 oz. cooked weight	250	—
Rice, 1.5 cups cooked	300	65
Broccoli, 1 cup	50	10
Dinner rolls, 2 whole wheat (2 oz.)	200	40
Snack:	**360**	**70**
Banana, 1 medium (4 oz.)	100	25
Sherbet, 1 cup	260	45
TOTAL	**3,200**	**563**

Do not worry that you will gain weight and "get fat" during this week of tapering and eating. The extra carbohydrate calories you consume (or rather, that you do not expend) will be stored as glycogen in your liver and muscles. During the weeks and months of athletic training, your muscles have increased their capacity to store glycogen. Your goal with tapering is to fill these

3,400 Total Calories	Calories	Carbs. (g)
Breakfast:	**800**	**152**
Oatmeal, 1 cup dry	300	55
Milk, 16 oz.	200	25
Raisins, ¼ cup	130	30
Brown sugar, 1.5 Tbsp	50	12
Apple juice, 8 oz.	120	30
Lunch:	**980**	**155**
Sub sandwich roll, 6-inch	320	60
Lean meat, 4 oz. cooked weight	200	—
Fruit yogurt, 8 oz.	240	40
Grape juice, 12 oz.	220	55
Snack:	**480**	**103**
Fig Newtons, 6	330	65
Jelly beans, 15 large (1.5 oz.)	150	38
Dinner:	**940**	**188**
Spaghetti, 2 cups cooked	400	80
Spaghetti sauce, 1 cup	250	40
Italian bread, 2 slices (1.5 oz.)	150	30
Root beer, 12 oz.	140	38
Snack:	**200**	**48**
Canned peaches in syrup, 1 cup	200	48
TOTAL	**3,400**	**646**

1 cup = 240 milliliters; 1 tablespoon = 15 milliliters; 1 ounce = 28 grams or 30 milliliters

Nutrition information from food labels, USDA National Nutrient Database (online), and J. Pennington, 2004, Bowes & Church's Food Values of Portions Commonly Used, 18th ed. (Philadelphia: Lippincott, Williams & Wilkins)

large stores to their capacity by eating a carbohydrate-rich, healthful diet. This assures that you will have a full tank of fuel for your event. Now if you are weighing yourself, be forewarned that the scale will go up. This is good! It means you have stored glycogen. For every ounce (28 grams) of carbohydrate stored in your body, you store about three ounces (85 grams) of water.

This can translate into three to four pounds (1.5 to 2 kilograms) by the end of your tapering week.

Be sure that you are *carbo*-loading, not *fat*-loading. In the name of carbo-loading, some riders eat bread slathered with butter, cheesy/creamy pasta dishes, baked potatoes glistening with butter and sour cream, and rich ice cream. These fatty foods fill the stomach and the fat cells but leave the muscles poorly fueled. This is because dietary fat is not converted to glycogen. If the fat you eat is not needed immediately for energy (for instance, if you will head to the sofa or to bed after eating), it is stored as body fat. The same is true for alcohol. And contrary to popular notion, most of the calories in beer and wine come from alcohol, not carbohydrates. Your best bet for carbo-loading is to trade extra fat and alcohol calories for extra carbohydrate calories:

Instead of:	Calories	Choose:	Calories
1 roll with butter	200	2 plain rolls or	200
		1 roll with honey or jelly	200
1 cup pasta with oil, cream, or cheese sauce; cheese ravioli, lasagna, or tortellini	300-350	1½ cups pasta with tomato sauce	300-350
1 scoop ice cream	200	2 scoops low-fat frozen yogurt	200
Bottle of beer or glass of wine	150	1 cup cranberry juice	150
		or 2 cups fat-free milk	150
		or a can of cola	150
Baked potato with butter/sour cream	300	Baked potato with ketchup or salsa plus extra dinner roll	300

Do not overlook protein-rich foods the days before your event. Endurance athletes burn a little protein for energy and your body requires protein on a daily basis. It is important to eat an appropriate amount of protein every day (see chapter 6). Eat a small serving of low-fat protein as an accompaniment to your meal (do not make protein the main focus), such as poached eggs, yogurt, milk, turkey, fish, or chicken, or plant proteins such as beans, lentils, or tofu (as your intestines can tolerate them).

THE CYCLIST'S FOOD GUIDE: FUELING FOR THE DISTANCE

• **THE DAY BEFORE THE EVENT**—By now, you may have gained about three to four pounds, but don't panic. This weight gain reflects water weight and indicates that your muscles are well-fueled with glycogen. Today is the day to maintain these glycogen stores by enjoying wholesome, carbohydrate-based meals. Don't feel you need to load up with a huge pasta dinner. Instead, why not enjoy a substantial carbohydrate-rich meal earlier in the day at breakfast or lunch? This allows more time for the food to digest and move through your system. You'll be better off eating a little bit more than less on the day before an event. But don't gorge either. Learning the right balance takes practice. Let each preparatory race and long ride be opportunities to learn.

Be sure to drink extra fluids, including water, juices, and soft drinks, to make sure you are fully hydrated. Your urine should be pale yellow and of significant quantity. Abstain from too much wine, beer, and other alcoholic beverages because they can have a dehydrating effect and do not contribute significant carbohydrates.

• **THE MORNING OF THE EVENT**—With luck, you will wake up to a clear, crisp day that makes you want to jump out of bed and jump onto your bike! Before embarking upon your day's task, be sure to eat breakfast. It is the most important meal of the day (see chapter 2). One of the biggest nutritional mistakes made by novice riders and racers is eating too little beforehand.

As we have mentioned, on your event day be sure to eat only foods and fluids that you have tried and that have worked for you in training. This will help you to avoid unwanted stomach ailments and other problems during your ride. If you are used to having a bagel and juice for breakfast, don't feast on pancakes the morning of the ride only to discover that they settle like a lead balloon. You should have learned during training which foods in which amounts your body tolerates before riding. Some cyclists can eat a light breakfast the hour before an event. Some bring food with them to the starting line. Others want six hours for their stomach to empty; they have learned they feel best if they wake up at 4 a.m., eat a bowl of oatmeal, and then go back to bed.

Drink plenty of familiar fluids the morning of the event: water, sports drinks, juices, and soft drinks. Water takes 45 to 90 minutes to move through your system, so you can drink several glasses up to two hours before the ride and have time to urinate the excess. Top-off your tank with one more glass 5 to 15 minutes before you start riding.

If you are used to having coffee or tea in the morning, do so on event day as well. Some riders drink coffee for mental stimulation or for its laxative effect. Others prefer to abstain because they are already nervous and jittery and have no need for an added buzz. Drinking a mug of hot coffee, warm water with lemon, or hot tea with breakfast stimulates the colon so that you may have a bowel movement, something you might want to achieve before you leave home. Pack extra water, sports drink, latte, juice, soda, or whatever beverages you like (and have tried in training) so they will be available for you at the event. Choose what is best for your body, and do what you normally do for your training rides.

● **DURING THE EVENT**—Your job during the ride or race is to prevent dehydration and maintain a normal blood sugar level. Both are essential to maximize your enjoyment and performance during the ride you have been training long and hard for. These topics are discussed in chapters 8, 10, and 11. Remember, do nothing new, special, or different during your event. Stick with what has worked for you and what is familiar to you in your training rides. That is, stick with the tried-and-true, and you will have an enjoyable, well-fueled, and successful ride.

● **SUMMARY**—By event day, you should be well-trained. You should have not only strong muscles but also a strong knowledge of the foods and fluids you need to fuel those muscles. Knowing you are nutritionally prepared, you need not fear that you will tire prematurely. Instead, you can focus on the day's job: completing the distance strongly and successfully with energy to spare!

• As part of your daily training program, you should eat a carbohydrate-rich diet every day. Choose wholesome grain products, such as pasta, rice, whole-grain bread, or cereal as the foundation of every meal, along with plenty of fruits and vegetables and smaller amounts of protein and dairy products.

- For competitive endurance events lasting longer than 90 minutes, load your muscles and liver with glycogen days before the event by tapering your training and eating your usual high-carbohydrate sports diet.
- Maintain optimal hydration status by drinking water, juice, soda, or sports drinks. Urine should be pale yellow and of significant quantity.
- To avoid nutrition mistakes and unwanted surprises, try nothing new on event day.

Words of wisdom from other cyclists... ━━━━━━━━━━━

"I used to think, 'I have big races coming up. I have to get stronger, so I will ride longer and harder right before a race.' Big mistake! I would feel extremely fatigued at the starting line. Now, I taper my training to half my usual, starting one week before an event. I am relaxed and ready to go."
Kate Riedell, Fairfield, CT

"To prepare for racing, my most important day is two days before an event. I start hydrating well. I make sure I get to bed early. I pay close attention to my sports diet, and either take the day off or do a very easy workout."
MaryAnn Martinez, Concord, MA

CHAPTER 14

Tips for the Traveling Cyclist

RAVELING TO ANOTHER CITY, STATE, OR COUNTRY TO PARTICIPATE IN a long ride or race presents its nutritional challenges. The same goes for bike touring. Your food routine is disrupted. You may not have access to foods you are used to eating. And you are confronted with rich temptations that lurk in every restaurant, cafe, and pushcart. All too often you can get sidetracked by the confusion and excitement of being in a new place.

Consuming food or drink that has not been part of your training diet can lead to a number of problems: constipation, stomach upset, diarrhea, gas, dehydration, and too few calories, any of which can hinder your performance and enjoyment on the ride. There is delicious food to be eaten all over the world, and for hungry bikers, it can be tempting to nosh on local fare before or during a ride. If you have an iron stomach, go ahead and enjoy. But for those who want to play it safe and avoid intestinal problems, stick to what you know. You'll ride with confidence knowing that you have eaten your usual sports food, not something new or different that may torment you during the ride!

On a routine day, staying hydrated can be a challenge, but maintaining optimal hydration is even trickier when you are traveling. For one thing, you are not in your usual environment, so water may be inaccessible or you may forget to drink regularly. Plus, riding in a different climate and/or altitude requires you to be even more vigilant about your hydration status. Climate affects your body's cooling system. You may get hotter and require more fluid to stay hydrated. In hot, dry climates, you may sweat more but not realize it because the sweat rapidly evaporates. At higher elevations breathing rate usually increases, resulting in greater water evaporation from your lungs. Stay on top of your hydration by drinking often, taking water with you wherever you go, and drinking on a schedule. (For more on hydration, see chapter 8.)

One key to successfully selecting a top-notch sports diet when you travel is to bring your usual foods and liquids with you. Do not assume the event, venue, hotel, or roadside store will supply you with what you are accustomed to eating. Many organized rides feature food stops along the way that offer anything from familiar peanut butter and jelly to unfamiliar sports bars, gels, and drinks. If you want to try a new sports food or drink, save it for a training ride close to home. This way, you won't risk jeopardizing your comfort and performance by experiencing heartburn, indigestion, or worse.

When traveling, it is easy to become sidetracked by the confusion and excitement of being in a new place. Fight the urge to do too much exploring the day before the ride. Better yet, save the sightseeing and exotic food noshing until after the ride. Allow your muscles to get fully fueled by putting your feet up and resting your legs. Relax with some juices and other tried-and-true carbohydrates, and visualize yourself completing the distance smoothly, strongly, and successfully.

Here are a few tips to help you accommodate a carbohydrate-rich sports diet into your traveling routine.

Breakfast:
- At a restaurant, order pancakes, French toast, whole-wheat toast, bagels, or bran muffins. Add honey, jam, or maple syrup for extra carbohydrates. Hold the butter or request that it is served on the side so that you can better control the amount of saturated fat in your meal, or use peanut butter instead.
- Limit cheese omelets, fried potatoes, bacon, biscuits, sausages and other fatty, greasy foods that will leave your muscles unfueled.
- Most restaurants offer cold cereals, oatmeal, and fat-free or low-fat milk, if this is what you prefer in the morning. Add banana, raisins, or brown sugar for more carbohydrates.

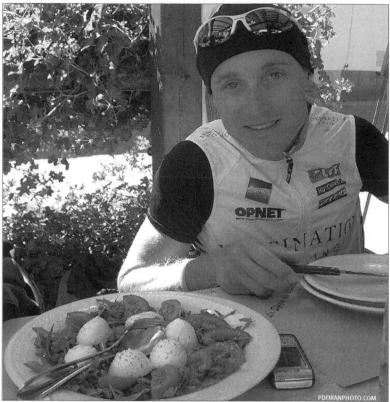

When touring in foreign countries, hungry cyclists have the opportunity to enjoy the local food—and plenty of it!

- Order a large orange juice or tomato juice. This helps compensate for a potential lack of fruits or vegetables in the other meals.
- For a hotel stay or for early morning events, pack your own cereal, banana or raisins, bowl or cup, spoon, and bottled juice. Bring powdered milk, a milk box (Parmalat or other shelf-stable milk or soymilk), or a cooler with cold milk or yogurt. Or, buy low-fat milk at a local convenience store.

Lunch:

- Find a deli or sandwich shop that offers bagels or wholesome breads. Request a sandwich that emphasizes the bread rather than the filling (preferably lean beef, turkey, ham, or chicken). Limit mayonnaise, butter, or oil-based dressing, and add tomatoes and lettuce. Add more carbohydrates with chocolate low-fat milk, juice, fruit, pretzels, or yogurt (buy these at a convenience store if the deli doesn't have them).

- At fast-food restaurants, limit the burgers, fried fish, fried chicken, and French fries. They contain a great deal of fat, primarily unhealthful trans or saturated fat. You'll get more carbohydrates by sticking to the spaghetti, baked potatoes, chili, or thick-crust pizza.
- Request thick-crust pizza with vegetable toppings rather than thin-crust pizza with pepperoni or sausage. Blot off the excess grease from the top of the pizza with a few napkins.
- Many supermarkets have salad and soup bars, deli or sandwich counters, and hot meal sections that offer a variety of healthful and tasty food. While you're there, pick up some yogurt, fruit, juice, bagels, or fig bars for snacks later on.
- At a salad bar, generously pile on the high-carbohydrate items such as chickpeas or other beans, fruit, and starchy vegetables like beets, carrots, and peas. Take plenty of bread. But don't fat-load on butter, salad dressings, and mayonnaise-smothered pasta and potato salads.
- A baked potato is a super choice if you request it plain rather than drenched with butter, sour cream, and cheese toppings. For moistness, mash the potato with some milk (order a glass of milk with your meal), add a tablespoon of sour cream (request it on the side), or top it with ketchup or salsa.
- Choose hearty soups, such as split pea, bean, minestrone, lentil, or noodle, accompanied by crackers, bread, a plain bagel, or an English muffin. Avoid cream-based soups like fish chowders, bisques, and cheese soups, which offer more fat and less carbohydrate.
- Juices and soft drinks are rich in carbohydrates, but juices are nutritionally preferable for vitamin C, potassium, and wholesome goodness.
- Consider ordering a glass of low-fat or fat-free milk or chocolate milk with your lunch. Often, milk is overlooked as source of carbohydrates, not to mention calcium and protein.
- Forgo restaurant food and bring your own lunch fixings. Fill a cooler with: turkey slices or homemade tuna salad, sliced low-fat cheese, peanut butter, baby carrots, cherry tomatoes, apples, low-fat milk, juice, yogurts, and grapes. Pack a loaf of whole-wheat bread or a package of multi-grain bagels, and oatmeal-raisin cookies or dried fruit.

Dinner:

- Check the restaurant beforehand to see if it offers abundant carbohydrates (pasta, baked potatoes, rice, steamed vegetables, salad bar, homemade bread, fruit, and juice) and lower-fat options such as broiled, grilled, or roasted fish, poultry, or meats. Inquire how dishes are made. Request they be prepared with minimal fat.
- Eat the breads and rolls either plain or with jelly or honey. Replace the butter calories with high-carbohydrate choices: another slice of bread, a second potato, soup and crackers, juice, sherbet, or frozen yogurt.
- When ordering salads, always request the dressing be served on the side. Otherwise, you may get as many as 400 calories of oil or mayonnaise, fatty foods that fill your stomach but leave your muscles unfueled.

Snacks:

- Pack your own snacks: pumpernickel bagels, corn muffins, banana bread, rolls, pretzels, fig bars, graham crackers, oatmeal-raisin cookies, granola, oranges, raisins, dried or fresh fruit, and juice boxes.
- Buy wholesome snacks at a convenience or grocery store. Good choices include: trail mix made with nuts and dried fruits, banana, raisins, nuts, cereal bar or granola bar, yogurt, 100% vegetable or fruit juice, bagel or hot pretzel, energy bar, slice of thick-crust pizza, small sandwich, or cup of soup.

- **SUMMARY**—Traveling to cycling events and cycle touring present nutritional challenges. Not only is your usual food routine disrupted, you are likely to be confronted with rich and tasty temptations that haven't been part of your training diet.
- Stick to tried-and-true foods and fluids that you know will settle well and not upset your digestive system. That way you'll have no unwanted surprises to ruin your ride.
- If you have any doubts about the availability of familiar foods, plan ahead and bring some safe foods with you.
- Pay particular attention to maintaining your hydration by drinking frequently and bringing water with you. It's easy to get sidetracked and forget to drink when you are traveling and having fun.

- If you want to try a new sports food or drink, try it on a training ride close to home and not on an important ride. This way, you won't risk jeopardizing your comfort and performance. For the same reason, save the exotic food sampling and local foodstuffs for after the ride.

Words of wisdom from other cyclists... ━━━━━━━━━━━━━━

"In my racing days, we saved money when traveling by never eating breakfast out. We'd eat in the hotel room— bagels, fruit, and cereal either brought from home or purchased at a store the night before. My teammate always brought hard-boiled eggs from home. They traveled well in the cooler. "
Karen Mackin, Acton, MA

"Before driving to the start of a ride, I pack plenty of fluids in a cooler, including my recovery drinks. They stay cold in the car while I'm biking and are a ready and waiting for me at the end when I'm tired and thirsty."
Jessica Truslow, Arlington, MA

"Before the evening start of a 600K brevet, I ate at a restaurant that served trendy "raw" vegan food, something new for me. It tasted great, but about an hour later my stomach started a most frightening rumbling and a bit later I sought refuge behind a container trailer. It was not a great way to start the ride."
Elmar Stefke, Berkeley, CA

CHAPTER 15

Calculating Your Calorie Needs

YOU MAY NOT THINK YOU COME CLOSE TO NEEDING THE 6,000 OR more calories that a Tour De France rider needs a day during the famous 21-day stage race. But if you are an active cyclist, you certainly require plenty of calories. Cyclists burn many calories because the sport involves continual hard effort sustained for hours at a time most days of the week. You burn on average 400 to 700 calories an hour on the bike, so you can easily rackup a thousand (or a couple thousand) calories during an afternoon training ride. Long-distance and touring cyclists who ride all day long for days, weeks, or months at a time, can indeed burn as many calories as a racer in the Tour. Physical demands of cycling aside, you are constantly burning calories. You need calories simply to exist: to breathe, blink, pump blood, and yes, to click the television remote control on recovery days.

● **COUNTING CALORIES**—Most cyclists can naturally regulate a proper calorie intake and have little need to count calories. They eat when they are hungry and stop when they are content. Others have lost touch with their body's ability to regulate an appropriate food intake—they may deny themselves food when they are hungry (as often happens with reducing diets), but then overeat later on. If that is your case, keep reading!

Counting calories can help erratic eaters and dieters to get in touch with appropriate portion sizes and acknowledge how much better they feel when they are appropriately fed. Once educated about how much is appropriate to eat, they can then learn how to regulate their food intake without counting calories. Calorie

Here are approximate calorie needs for cyclists of different weights who are moderately active throughout the day*:

Weight	Approximate calorie needs for:	(ride speeds are not with drafting)		
lbs (kg)	daily living	+ 2-hour ride at 11 mph (18 km/hr)	+ 2-hour ride at 15 mph (24 km/hr)	+ 2-hour ride at 18 mph (29 km/hr)
120 (55)	1,800	+600 = 2,400	+ 1,100 = 2,900	+1,320 = 3,120
140 (64)	2,100	+700 = 2,800	+ 1,280 = 3,380	+1,540 = 3,640
160 (73)	2,400	+800 = 3,200	+ 1,460 = 3,860	+1,750 = 4,150
180 (82)	2,700	+900 = 3,600	+ 1,640 = 4,340	+1,970 = 4,670

*Calorie expenditure information from Ainsworth et al., 2000.

information can also help touring cyclists, randonneurs, and other long-distance cyclists who may not feel hungry while riding to fuel themselves adequately on long rides. (See page 146 for estimating your calorie needs.)

● **HONOR HUNGER**—More important than counting calories is to simply listen to hunger signals: inability to focus, fatigue, bad mood, thoughts about food. Stomach growling tells you that you have become too hungry; you should eat before you reach this stage. Generally, the more you exercise, the hungrier you will get. Whereas most cyclists honor their hunger by refueling with wholesome meals, others feel confused by hunger and sometimes even feel guilty that they are always eager to eat.

Hunger is not bad or wrong. It is simply your body's way of telling you it needs more fuel; you should respond appropriately by eating. You should not spend your day feeling hungry, weak, and tired, even if you are trying to lose weight (see chapter 16). If your 8 a.m. breakfast leaves you hungry earlier than 11 a.m., your breakfast contained too few calories. You need to eat either a bigger breakfast or a midmorning snack. If you are hungry all afternoon, starving by dinnertime, and overeating in the evening, you are not eating enough during the day.

Cyclists need good food on a regular schedule. Eat at least every four hours during the day. Allot about one-fourth of your day's calories for each section of the day (morning, midday, afternoon, and evening). So, halfway through your active day

By using the following formula, you can *roughly estimate* your personal calorie needs and gain a perspective on how to balance calories eaten versus calories expended. These guidelines do not address the needs of each individual. For personalized calorie information, you should meet with a registered dietitian who specializes in sports nutrition. To contact a sports nutritionist in your area, use the referral networks at www.eatright.org or www.SCANdpg.org.

1. To estimate your resting metabolic rate, that is, the amount of calories you need to simply breathe, pump blood, and be alive, multiply your weight by 10 calories per pound (or 22 calories per kilogram). (If you are significantly overweight, use a weight that is halfway between your desired weight and your current weight.) So, if you weigh 150 pounds (70 kilograms), you need approximately 1,500 calories simply to do nothing all day except exist:

   150 pounds x 10 calories/pound = 1,500 calories

2. Add more calories for activities of daily living *apart from your riding* and other purposeful exercise (see note below). Add:
   * 30 to 40 percent if you are mostly sedentary (sitting, typing, reading, resting, or taking it easy to recover from a ride);
   * 50 percent if you are moderately active (frequently standing and walking, doing household chores, moving often throughout the day); or
   * 60 to 70 percent or more if you are mostly or very active (sitting very little, working/walking on your feet most of the day).

If you weigh 150 pounds (70 kilograms) and are moderately active when you are not riding, you would add 50 percent to your resting metabolic rate (1,500 calories), or 750 calories, for activities of daily living. So, you may need 2,200 calories total in a day without riding:

   1,500 calories + 50% (or 750 calories) = 2,250 (let's say 2,200) calories a day
   without riding

Note: *For long-distance riders, the number of calories used for activities of daily living may actually be very small (because they are riding for most of the day and because they tend to be sedentary once they're off the bike). So when calculating your calorie needs for long-ride days, use a lower activity level so that you do not overestimate the total number of calories you burn in a day.*

3. Now, add more calories for your riding and other purposeful exercise. Refer to the chart on page 150. If you weigh 150 pounds (70 kilograms) and you ride consistently hard at 15 miles per hour without drafting for 1.5 hours, you burn approximately 1000 calories while riding. This brings your day's total calorie needs to approximately 3,200 calories:

- 150 pounds x 4.5 calories/pound/hour (see chart, page 150) = 675 calories/hour
- 675 calories/hour x 1.5 hour = 1,013 calories for the ride (let's say 1,000)
- 1,000 calories + 2,200 calories = 3,200 total calories/day with 1.5 hours of riding.

4 If you want to lose weight, subtract approximately 20 percent of your total calorie needs. If you want to gain, add 20 percent. If your daily calorie needs are 3,200 on ride days and you want to lose weight, subtract 600 calories or so from 3,200. This gives you a total of 2,600 calories a day to lose weight. On rest days, you may want just as many calories because your muscles need carbs to refuel.

3,200 calories −20% (or roughly 600 calories) = 2,600 calories per day
for weight loss on ride days

(Refer to chapters 16, 17, and 18 for more guidance on body weight.)

5. Finally, divide your day's calories budget evenly into three or four parts of the day: morning, noon/afternoon, and evening. Using our example, a 150-pound cyclist who is not trying to lose weight, would have a daily calorie budget that may look like this:

Meal	Calories Ride days	Calories Off Season
3 meals per day:		
Breakfast/snack	1,000	700
Lunch/snack	1,000	800
Dinner/snack	1,000	700
During 1.5 hours riding	+200-300	
Total	**3,200**	**2,200**
4 meals per day:		
Breakfast	800	600
Lunch	700	500
Lunch #2	700	500
Dinner	700	600
During 1.5 hours riding	+200-300	
Total	**3,200**	**2,200**

On ride days you may not feel hungry enough to eat this much, and on rest days you may be ravenous and need to eat more to refuel your muscles. Remember to listen to your appetite: eat when hungry and stop when content.

6. Read food labels to become familiar with the calorie content of the foods you commonly eat and then balance your calorie budget according to the rules for a well-balanced diet.

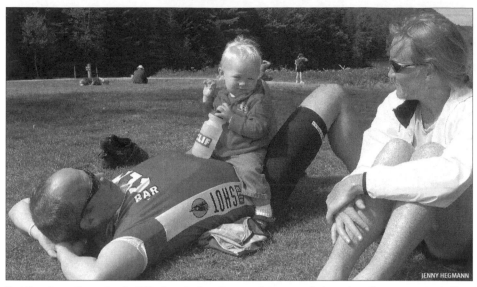

Toddlers have the natural ability to eat when they are hungry and stop when they are content. Many adults have lost this ability, but can relearn how to eat appropriately.

you should have consumed half of your day's calories. This approach is particularly helpful to cyclists who feel tired or hungry all the time, lack energy for workouts, or are trying to change their weight.

It's OK to satisfy your calorie needs with three, four, or more meals a day, depending on your appetite and preference. Just eat evenly on a schedule. If you like to eat multiple mini-meals, for example, you can eat a light breakfast early and then eat a second breakfast midmorning to satisfy your energy needs. Eat lunch (the second-most-important meal of your sports diet) around noon and then a second lunch later in the afternoon. Morning riders need a hearty lunch to refuel their muscles; afternoon riders need a respectable lunch for their after-work ride. Finally, enjoy a wholesome dinner in the evening to refuel from your busy day. If you won't be home for your usual dinnertime, then plan to eat a substantial part of your dinner calories early (in the afternoon).

If this sounds like a lot of daytime food to you, you may be eating backwards. That is, if you do most of your eating in the evening and battle hunger all day, stop! Shift some of those evening calories to the daytime, so you will have more energy during the day when you need it most. Your workouts will be

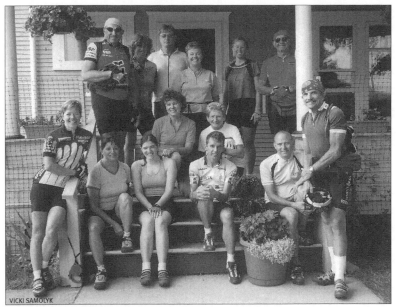

Cyclists come in all ages, sizes, and shapes and have different calorie requirements. But by honoring hunger, each cyclist can fuel optimally for high energy.

stronger, you will feel more energetic and awake, and you won't be distracted by constant hunger.

● **DO I REALLY NEED THAT MANY CALORIES???**—Keep in mind that the precise number of calories burned by an individual can be measured only with special metabolic equipment in a well-controlled lab setting. Calorie expenditure depends on many factors, including your fitness level, age, gender, and, of course, how hard you ride. You burn many more calories when you ride uphill, with a heavy load, or into the wind than when you ride downhill, unencumbered, or with a tailwind. Racers know that they can conserve energy by drafting behind other riders in the pack. Also, body position affects how many calories you burn: Standing on the pedals burns more calories than sitting with hands on brake hoods, which burns more calories than sitting, tucked in the aero position.

On hard-ride days, you burn many more calories than usual. This can present a dilemma: When do you eat those extra calories? If you are eating appropriately, the 200 or so calories you consume before and during each hour of riding plus your recovery meal will help you meet your calorie needs on ride

● ENERGY EXPENDITURE OF BICYCLING AND OTHER ACTIVITIES

To estimate how many calories you use during an activity:

Take your weight and multiply it by the calories used per hour of activity. Then multiply that number by how many hours (or fractions of hours) during which you maintained the activity. For example, a 150-pound (70-kilogram) cyclist who rides at an average pace of 15 miles per hour (24 kilometers per hour) for 1.5 hour alone (not drafting) will burn approximately 1000 calories during that activity:

150 lb x 4.5 cal/lb/hr = 675 cal/hr; 675 cal/hr x 1.5 hr = 1013 calories

Bicycling: *Calories used per pound or kilogram of body weight per hour*

Speed	Description	cal/lb/hr	cal/kg/hr
11 mph (18 km/hr)	leisure, slow, light effort	2.5	6
13 mph (21 km/hr)	leisure, moderate effort	3.5	8
15 mph (24 km/hr)	racing or leisure, fast, vigorous effort	4.5	10
16-19 mph (26-31 km/hr)	racing, not drafting, fast	5.5	12
>19 mph (31 km/hr)	racing, drafting, very fast	5.5	12
> 20 mph (32 km/hr)	racing, not drafting, very fast	7.5	16
unspecified	mountain, cross, or BMX biking	4	8.5

Other Activities: *Calories used per pound or kilogram of body weight per hour*

Description	cal/lb/hr	cal/kg/hr
Hockey, field or ice	3.5	8
Lying awake or sitting quietly, watching TV, reading	0.5	1
Running, 6 mph (10 km/hr)	4.5	10
Running, 8 mph (13 km/hr)	6	13.5
Running, 10 mph (16 km/hr)	7.5	16
Skiing, cross-country, 4-5 mph (6.5-8 km/hr), moderate effort	3.5	8
Skiing, cross-country, 5-8 mph (8-13 km/hr), vigorous effort	4	9
Skiing, cross-country, >8 mph (13 km/hr), racing, hard effort	6.5	14
Skiing, downhill, moderate effort	2.5	6
Skiing, downhill, vigorous effort, racing	3.5	8
Sleeping	0.4	0.9
Soccer, casual, general	3	7
Stretching, Hatha yoga	1	2.5
Swimming, freestyle, fast, vigorous effort	4.5	10
Swimming, freestyle, slow, moderate effort	3	7
Walking, level surface, 3 to 4 mph (4.5 to 6.5 km/hr)	1.5-2.5	3.5-5
Walking, uphill, 3 mph (4.5 km/hr)	2.5	6
Weight lifting (free, Nautilus- or Universal-type), body building, vigorous effort	2.5	6
Weight lifting (free, Nautilus- or Universal-type), body building, light or moderate effort	1.5	3

Adapted from Ainsworth BE, et al, 2000.

days. In addition, riding makes you hungry (sooner or later, if not during or immediately afterward), so you will naturally want to eat more on that day or the next day. If your weight is not changing and you feel energetic overall, you are meeting your calorie requirements. Eating for riding is discussed more thoroughly in chapters 10 and 11.

• SUMMARY—

- Hungry cyclists need good, wholesome food on a regular schedule so they can enjoy an even flow of energy throughout the day. You should plan to eat at least every four hours, if not more often. Honor hunger by eating nourishing foods when your body requests fuel.
- Knowing how many calories you need can help you to plan big enough meals at breakfast and lunch, so you avoid being hungry all day long.
- Fueling before, during, and after riding will help you to meet the caloric demands of cycling.
- Feeling hungrier on the days you ride, or the day after, is normal and allows you to eat enough to support your training and refueling program.

Words of wisdom from other cyclists... ▬▬▬▬▬▬▬▬▬▬▬▬▬

"As director of the Pan-Mass Challenge, I have noticed that some cyclists, often women, have a hard time eating enough to support their riding. They think food will make them fat. But they need to realize that if they don't eat, they won't perform."
Billy Starr, Boston, MA

"The worst nutritional mistake I have made was assuming biking allowed me to eat whatever I wanted, and not gain weight."
Rich Lesnik, San Francisco, CA

"Before our Trans-America tour, many in the group assumed they would lose weight effortlessly. The opposite actually happened. People gained weight. Some of the weight was muscle, but some of it was fat. We enjoyed eating when we weren't biking and we could too easily rationalize that extra piece of pie or milk shake."
Candice Crowell, Georgetown, MA

CHAPTER 16

How to Lose Weight and Have Energy to Ride

EXERCISE BURNS CALORIES, AND THAT IS ONE OF THE REASONS WHY people bike, run, and enjoy other forms of physical activity. Consistent exercise helps them manage their weight and allows more freedom with eating. But for many active people weight remains a significant issue. There are plenty of cyclists who are in a constant battle with their weight and feel frustrated that they just can't seem to shed those final few pounds. Inevitably, the first words they say are, "I know what to do to lose weight. I just can't do it." They think they should follow a strict diet with rigid rules and regulations. Wrong. Diets don't work. If diets did work, everyone who has ever dieted would be as thin as desired. The key to losing weight is to stop thinking about going on a diet and start learning how to eat healthfully.

● **HOW MUCH IS OKAY TO EAT?**—To determine just how much you can appropriately eat, refer to the previous chapter. Note that your body requires a large amount of energy to simply exist—to pump blood, breathe, produce urine, and grow hair. Also note that you deserve to eat those maintenance calories even if you are injured and unable to ride.

An appropriate reducing diet knocks off only 20 percent (or less) of your calorie needs. To do this, you need to know how many calories your body requires and how many calories you're eating. Let's take a look at Jane, a 5-foot 2-inch, 120-pound (157-cm, 55-kg) graduate student, who wanted to lose "those last five pounds." She biked for an hour on most days to relieve stress and to "burn fat." She required about 2,200 to 2,300 calories to maintain her weight:

- 1,200 calories for her resting metabolic rate (10 calories per pound x 120 pounds) +
- 600 calories for general activity (50% x 1,200 calories) +
- 500 calories for an hour of cycling (4.0 calories/pound/hour x 120 pounds).

To appropriately lose weight, she needed to cut her total calorie intake by 20 percent (about 400 to 500 calories), leaving her with 1,800 calories for her diet plan.

To Jane, 1,800 sounded like too many calories. She exclaimed, "I could never eat that much; I'd gain weight! If I can't lose weight eating only 1,000 calories a day, how could I possibly lose weight eating 1,800 calories? My metabolism is so slow..."

Although Jane challenged the calorie recommendations, Nancy suggested that she keep an open mind. The latest research on athletes' calorie needs suggests that very few athletes actually do have slow metabolisms. Researchers even have studied active people like Jane who claim to maintain weight despite eating next to nothing. When carefully monitored, these women burned the calories one would expect based on standard calculations. Their metabolisms were fine, but they had problems acknowledging—

- how inactive they were apart from their purposeful exercise, and
- how much food they actually ate. Their mindless nibbles on bagels, apples, rice cakes, and broken cookies added up!

For more information, refer to *Slow Metabolism Woes* on page 164.

Because Jane claimed she ate far less than her peers, she needed to heighten her awareness of her food intake by keeping food records to track everything she ate. Food records can be extremely useful to help you understand your eating habits. You might notice that you:

- Eat when reading and don't even notice the portion.
- Eat too little at breakfast and lunch, only to overeat at night.
- Diet Monday through Thursday, then splurge on weekends.

Research indicates that keeping accurate food records can help people lose weight. By knowing what and when you eat, why you eat, and where you eat, you can take the necessary steps to eat 20 percent less, an appropriate reducing diet.

● **FIVE KEYS TO SUCCESSFUL WEIGHT REDUCTION—**If you want to lose weight healthfully and keep it off, we suggest you estimate your energy needs (see the previous chapter) and follow these five recommendations.

Key #1. Eat enough. Don't get too hungry or you will blow your diet. Many weight-conscious cyclists try to eat as little as possible. That's a big mistake. Perhaps the following case study will help you understand why. Cindi thought skimping on food was a good way to diet and she felt frustrated by her lack of weight loss. She explained, "I have only coffee for breakfast. I exercise at lunchtime and then just eat a salad with cottage cheese. Nighttime is my trouble-time. I just cannot seem to stay away from the frozen yogurt. It seems the more I diet, the more weight I gain."

Clearly, *not eating* was Cindi's problem. Dieting and denial were getting her nowhere. She needed to accept that she is supposed to eat and to trust that appropriate eating will contribute to an appropriate weight.

In trying to stick to her bare-bones diet, Cindi's breakfast and lunch totaled less than a quarter of the 2,400 calories she required. It is no wonder that she lacked energy for her afternoon workouts and was starving by dinnertime! All too often, she would skip the workout and then eat everything in sight at night, only to get up the next morning with a food hangover. She would then vow to get back on her diet, skip breakfast, skimp on lunch, lack energy to enjoy exercise, and blow her diet again at night. Although Cindi deserved a lot of credit for having the willpower to survive the day on so few calories, her method was mistaken. Her diet was too strict.

If you, like Cindi, are trying to lose weight by eating as little as possible and exercising as hard as you can, remember that the less you eat, the more likely you are to blow your diet. Even if you can successfully restrict your intake, the less you eat, the more your body adjusts to having fewer calories. You will start to hibernate similar to what a bear does in winter when food is scarce. Your metabolic rate will drop to conserve calories and you will feel lethargic, cold, grumpy, and lack energy to pedal strongly through a workout. Why bother to eat next to nothing when you can lose weight with eating just 20 percent less than you need to maintain your weight?

Most female cyclists like Cindi who want to lose weight should follow 1,800- to 2,200-calorie (or greater) reduction diets, depending on how hard they train. Most male cyclists can lose weight eating 2,400 to 2,800 (or more) calories. This is far more than most 800- to 1,200-calorie diets that are designed for sedentary people who can get away with eating very little. You need a substantial amount of energy to fuel your muscles and have energy to enjoy your training.

Key #2. Be sure that you eat more during the day, so that you will be able to eat less (diet) at night. For an appropriate reducing program, divide your calories evenly throughout the day. Keep in mind that athletes tend to get hungry (and should

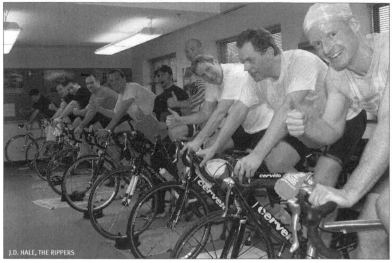

To avoid winter weight gain, stay active during the winter—and keep it fun!

eat) at least every four hours. A 150-pound (70-kilogram) cyclist who is on a 2,200-calorie reducing diet may plan the day as such:

Breakfast:	8 a.m.	600 calories
Lunch:	Noon	600 calories
Snack:	4 p.m.	400 calories
Ride 1 hour:	6 p.m.	
Dinner:	8 p.m.	600 calories

Your goal is to eat on a schedule to prevent yourself from getting too hungry.

Your training program may require creative meal scheduling if you exercise during meal times. For example, if you ride at 6 p.m., potentially at the height of your hunger, you might better enjoy your training if you eat part of your dinner beforehand. You could trade in your 200-calorie dinner potato for a pre-ride granola bar. Similarly, if you ride at 6 a.m., you might enjoy greater energy if you eat part of your breakfast beforehand, such as a slice of toast and a glass of juice, and then eat the rest afterwards to recover and to satisfy your hunger. As mentioned in chapter 10, you need to experiment with pre-exercise food to determine the right amount of calories to boost your energy without making you feel heavy and sluggish.

Some cyclists believe that riding "on empty," such as riding first thing in the morning without having eaten, burns more body fat than exercising well-fueled. While this is true, keep in mind that burning body fat does not equate to losing body fat. To have a net loss of body fat, you need to create and maintain a calorie deficit; you need to burn more calories than you consume over a period of days. People who exercise on empty usually do not achieve net fat loss because:

- they lack the energy for long, strong workouts, and end up burning fewer calories than someone who is properly fueled before exercise.
- they experience extreme hunger later on, which can lead to overeating calories later in the day.

Key #3. Eat an appropriate amount of fat. If you currently eat a high-fat diet filled with butter, mayonnaise, salad dressing, greasy meals, and rich desserts, you should cut back on these fattening foods. Excess dietary fat easily turns into excess body fat, if not cardiovascular disease.

Some of today's bikers try to totally avoid fat. They think that if they eat fat, they will instantly get fat. This is not always the case. Some fat in your food may actually help you lose weight. Take a look around and notice the number of trim cyclists whose diets include some fat. If you are trying to knock all the fat out of your diet, think again. Those who shun all fat:

- commonly feel hungry, denied, deprived,
- feel guilty when they inevitably "cheat" by eating fat, and
- eat an unbalanced diet that may be too low in protein and can hurt their performance.

One study showed that dieters who were instructed to eat 1,200 calories of a standard American (35-percent-fat) diet actually lost more body fat than the group who were instructed to eat 1,200 calories of a low-fat (20-percent-fat) diet (McManus et al. 2001). Why? Because the high-fat dieters were better able to comply with their regimen. Fat is helpful for dieters because it takes longer to digest and provides a nice feeling of satisfaction that can prevent you from searching through the kitchen for something tasty to eat. Fat is also needed to absorb certain vitamins.

You will enjoy more success with losing body fat if you give yourself a reasonable calorie and fat budget to spend on the foods that you want to eat. By choosing the 25-percent-fat diet that is described in chapter 7, you can add a little fat to each meal, provide your body with important nutrients, feel more satisfied, and be better able to stick to your diet. For generations, people have lost fat even though their diets included fat. You can too!

Key #4. You don't have to lose weight every day. Losing weight requires enough mental energy to tell yourself, "I'd rather be leaner than eat more calories." Some days you may lack that mental energy. For example, Jim, a stockbroker who wanted to lose five pounds before an Ironman triathlon, was stressed out by his demanding workload, training schedule, and family problems. Although he wanted to drop a few pounds, he lacked the mental energy he needed to cut calories. At the end of the day, he'd inevitably succumb to cookies, a nice reward for having survived the day. Jim needed to be reminded that he is only human, with a limited amount of mental and physical energy. Rather than getting mad at himself for eating cookies, he needed to accept the fact that he was stressed and in need of comfort. Like it or not, food provided that comfort.

Jim needed to let go of his current goal to lose fat and focus instead on maintaining his weight and fueling his muscles appropriately. Well-fueled muscles would enhance his training more than would poorly fueled muscles, especially if they were depleted from improper dieting. Jim reluctantly agreed to postpone his efforts to drop a few pounds.

Stressful times are often poor times to try to reduce body fat. Instead, you should focus on exercising regularly to help cope with stress and on eating healthfully to prevent the weight gain that sometimes occurs during stressful times. Note that cyclists who are both stressed and hungry can easily succumb to overeating, so it can be helpful to eat every four hours to keep your appetite at bay. Of course, no amount of food will solve any problem; it only adds to your feeling out of control.

Key #5. Have realistic weight goals. Weight is more than just a matter of willpower. Genetics plays a large role. If you are eating appropriately during the day, exercising regularly, eating

Food has many roles. It satisfies hunger, fuels muscles, is a pleasurable part of social gatherings and celebrations, rewards us at the end of a stressful day, and has a calming effect. If you tend to eat for reasons other than fuel, think HALT and ask yourself: Why do I want to eat? Is it because I am...
- **H**ungry?
- **A**ngry or Anxious?
- **L**onely?
- **T**ired?

If you are eating inappropriately, remember that no amount of food will solve any problem. Don't start eating if you know you will have problems stopping.

lighter at night, and waking up eager for breakfast but still have not lost body fat, perhaps you have an unrealistic goal. It is possible that you have no excess fat to lose and you are already very lean for your genetic blueprint.

Every body is different, but any body can be fit. Just take a look around at a bike race, tour, or ride and you will see all body types, from slight and sinewy to broad and muscle-bound. Like it or not, nature may want you to look more like a linebacker, than the narrow, lightweight racer you may wish to be.

Women cyclists in particular complain about their natural physiques, that biking makes their legs and butts bigger. Many wish their tight-fitting riding shorts better disguised their round hips and jiggly upper thighs. Earlier in this chapter, we mentioned Cindi, who was skimping on food, trying to eat as little as possible in her struggle to lose weight. Cindi was short and had big thighs, just like her mother and sisters. Although she put no effort into trying to grow taller, she obsessed about the fat on her thighs and spent lots of energy trying to reduce them.

Cindi needed to know that although she could remodel her body to a certain extent, she could not totally redesign it. Plain and simple, active people and athletes come in varying sizes and shapes. No single body type is right or wrong.

In order to determine an appropriate weight for your body, stop looking at the scale and start looking at your family.

Imagine yourself at a family reunion:
- How do you compare to other members of your family?
- Are you currently leaner than they are? fatter? the same?
- If leaner, are you straining to stay that way?
- If you are significantly leaner, you may already be underfat for your body.

Many people, cyclists and non-athletes alike, put their lives on hold, struggling to lose a final few pounds. Cindi would often say, grabbing her thighs, "I hate being seen in lycra shorts. But no matter how much I exercise, I can't get rid of these fat thighs. I must be doing something wrong." Cindi was simply trying to get to a weight that was abnormal for her genetics. She was already leaner than other members of her family.

She needed to understand the reason why women as compared to men have fat thighs: The fat in the hips, buttocks, and thighs is sex-specific. It is a storehouse of energy for potential pregnancy and breast-feeding and is supposed to be there. Just as women have breast tissue, women also have hip, buttock, and thigh tissue. Women have fatter derrieres and legs than men because women are women. Bicycling works the leg, gluteal, and hip muscles, so bikers should expect to gain muscle mass in those areas. But that doesn't change the fact that nature wants women to have some fat in those areas too. The result can be, yes, bigger thighs and butts, but also stronger muscular pistons to power you mile after mile. Cindi needed to accept the realities of being a woman and stop comparing herself to the magazine and catalog models who do indeed have rare physiques. For more on body image issues, see chapter 17.

If you are wasting time complaining about your body, keep in perspective:
- Life is a gift.
- Life is too short to be spent obsessing about food and weight.

Yes, you do want to be fit and healthy, but you need not strive to be sleek and skinny. The cost attached to achieving the perfect weight and the perfect body is often yo-yo dieting, poor nutrition, lack of energy to ride well, guilt for eating, a sense of failure that can play havoc with your self-esteem, and poor cycling performance. Love your body for what it is. Stop hating it for what it is not.

● **SUMMARY**—Food is fuel, energizing, and health-giving. You are supposed to eat even if you are trying to lose weight. Be realistic about your weight-loss expectations and remember:

- The best-fueled rider (not the thinnest rider) will likely be the strongest rider.
- You are supposed to eat even if you want to lose body fat. Deduct only 20 percent of your calorie budget, but do not starve yourself.
- You should eat during the day, and then diet at night. Early morning hunger is a sign you did not overeat the night before.
- Your diet should include a little bit of fat to keep you feeling satisfied, to help provide you with important nutrients, and to fuel long rides.
- Realize that you do not have to lose weight every day; stress-filled days can be for maintaining weight.
- Be realistic with your weight goals. You may have no weight to lose, according to your genetics.

Words of wisdom from other cyclists... ━━━━━━━━━━━━━━━

"I suggest that people spend a year trying all the different diets they can find. Then, after having no success at achieving their goals, they gradually modify their normal eating habits. There are no quick fixes for weight loss. Period. Show me a quick fix, and I will show you how you are hurting your body."
John Correia, San Diego, CA

"Over the winter off-season, my body fat increases somewhat. Come spring-time, I work to lose that extra body fat by cutting out refined carbs and sweets, like muffins and cookies, and eating more fruits, whole grains, and vegetables. That, combined with increased time on the bike, works for me."
MaryAnn Martinez, Concord, MA

"For a while I was trying to eat less so that I could weigh less, but I'd end up eating more and weighing more. I finally learned that if I eat sensibly—three meals per day—that my weight is fine. I feel better and exercise better."
Candace Strobach, Kinnelon, NJ

"I've finally learned to eat enough food during the day. I feel so much stronger all the time. I've actually lost weight while eating more food—but the secret is to eat more good food, not junk food."
Tracie Timothy, Salt Lake City, UT

CHAPTER 17

Dieting Gone Awry

ACTIVE PEOPLE OF ALL AGES AND ABILITIES APPRECIATE THE FITNESS, fun, and physical benefits that come with bicycling. Most cyclists have hearty, healthy appetites that support their exercise programs. Good nutrition helps them to:

- attain their goals of racing better, completing a tour, or enjoying a century ride,
- maintain energy to handle their fast-paced lifestyles,
- reduce their risk of injuries, and
- for women, ensure having regular menstrual periods.

But for some cyclists, eating presents challenges. Due to the prevailing myths that thinness contributes to both better performance and happiness, some cyclists consider food to be a fattening enemy rather than a friendly fuel. With the fear that eating meals will make them heavy and slow, they deny themselves permission to eat adequately. Appropriate meals are placed on hold until they lose those final few pounds and feel better about their weight.

Fueled by the "thinner is better" philosophy, cyclists who strive to be abnormally thin commonly pay a high price: eating disorders, poor nutrition, poorly fueled muscles, loss of menses (in women), stress fractures and other injuries, to say nothing of reduced stamina, endurance, and performance. In their over-concern about their weight they forget this formula for success:

appropriate eating + regular exercise = appropriate weight

Chapter 16 offers guidance about how to lose weight and maintain energy for riding. This chapter provides additional perspective to help resolve the food and weight obsessions of active men and women. The majority of this chapter is targeted to women, because women tend to be very weight-conscious. But if you are a man who struggles with food, the information will help you too.

● **WOMEN AND WEIGHT**—While both male and female cyclists can struggle with weight obsession, women clearly have more issues with food and weight than men have. Let's look at the possible explanations.

1. Women are supposed to have more body fat than men. Plain and simple, nature prescribes to women a certain amount of body fat that is essential for two reasons:
• to protect their ability to create and nourish healthy babies and
• to be a storehouse of calories for pregnancy and breast feeding.

This essential body fat is stored not only in the breasts but also in the hips, abdomen, buttocks, and upper legs, which explains why women have rounder hips and heavier thighs than most men. Women have almost three times as much essential body fat as men: 11 to 13 percent of a woman's body weight versus only 3 to 5 percent of a man's body weight is essential fat. Women who try to achieve the so-called "cut look" of male athletes create physiological turmoil and commonly pay the price by starving, bingeing, and obsessing about food in order to reach their desired image.

2. Women commonly target an unnatural weight. Women who try to get below their natural weight are the ones most likely to struggle with food and fight the battle with the bulge. Given that even some of those very lean and fast, front-of-the-pack women riders wish they could be lighter, it is not surprising that eating disorders abound. The majority of men, in comparison, seem to be more at peace with their natural weight and, consequently, at peace with food.

3. Women hold distorted body images. The Madison Avenue image that adorns every storefront and magazine ad leads us to believe that nature makes all women universally lean. Any aberration is thought to be a result of gluttony and lack of willpower. Wrong!

Nature makes us in different sizes and shapes, like it or not. If the cyclists who are discontent with their weight could only learn to accept and love their bodies, eating disorders would be rare. Take the story of a food-obsessed female cyclist. At 5-feet, 7-inches tall and 120 pounds (170 centimeters and 55 kilograms), she would lament, "I really wish I could weigh 110 pounds (50 kilograms)." A normal, healthy weight for a woman of her height is 135 pounds (61 kilograms)! She was unable to see that she was already very lean. She was training harder and harder to burn calories and lose body fat. Her training contrasted with that of other cyclists, commonly men, who train primarily to enhance performance, not to reshape their bodies.

● **SLOW METABOLISM WOES**—Frustration with inability to lose weight is common among people who claim they have a slow metabolism and eat less than they "deserve," given their rigorous daily exercise regimen. Perhaps you have heard your buddies express complaints similar to the following:

- I eat less than my friends but I still don't lose weight. There must be something wrong with my metabolism.
- I maintain weight on only 1,000 calories per day. I want to lose a few pounds, but I can't imagine eating any less.
- I ride every day and eat only one meal a day. I can't understand why I don't lose weight.

Is it true that some athletes are energy-efficient? Do they efficiently utilize every calorie they eat so they are able to maintain weight on fewer calories than their counterparts who seemingly eat more and unproductively burn them off? No.

According to Dr. Jack Wilmore, exercise physiologist at the University of Texas at Austin, the energy-efficient athlete does not exist. His research suggests that metabolic rate is closely tied to muscle mass. Dieters who overly restrict calories end up burning muscle tissue for energy and tend to have less muscle mass. Consequently, they require fewer calories. This is particularly true with women who constantly restrict their intake.

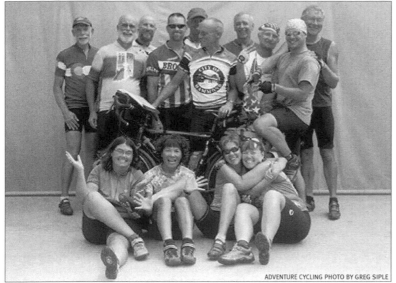

Enjoying group activities is difficult for cyclists who have a fearful relationship with food. Don't let food issues interfere with your quality of life!

Plain and simple, athletes who have well-developed muscles require more calories than those who have less muscle.

Other researchers believe that a slower metabolism may be nature's way to conserve calories when too few calories are being eaten. For instance, people who perceive themselves as being energy-efficient commonly complain about being cold all the time, feeling lethargic, and (in women) lacking regular menstrual cycles. These symptoms suggest that their diet is too meager to support normal body functions.

Your solution to the slow metabolism woes comes in finding the right amount of calories and nutrients to support a healthy weight for your body.

● **WOMEN AND AMENORRHEA**—If you are a cyclist or triathlete who previously had regular menstrual periods but have stopped menstruating, you are experiencing amenorrhea.

You may think your period stopped because you are too thin or are exercising too much, but that is not the case. There are plenty of very thin cyclists and elite athletes who do have regular menstrual periods, and studies have shown no body fat differences between athletes who regularly menstruate and those who don't (Sanborn et al. 2000).

Research suggests that amenorrhea is actually a nutritional problem and may be due to eating too little (Loucks 2001). Athletes with amenorrhea often struggle to maintain an unhealthy low weight, resulting in inadequate nutrition and consequently, loss of menses. Indeed, athletic amenorrhea is sometimes a red flag for an eating disorder. If the amenorrhea is caused by anorexia, it is a symptom of pain and unhappiness in your life.

If you feel you struggle harder than your counterparts to maintain your desired leanness, realize that you may be eating inadequately and putting yourself at risk for amenorrhea and all of its associated health problems. If you have stopped having regular menstrual periods, be sure to consult with your gynecologist for professional guidance.

● **HEALTH RISKS OF AMENORRHEA**—Although you may deem amenorrhea a desirable side effect of exercise because you no longer have to deal with the hassles and possible discomfort of monthly menstrual periods, amenorrhea can lead to undesirable problems that can interfere with your health and ability to perform at your best. These problems include:

- Almost a three times higher incidence of stress fractures
- Premature osteoporosis (weakening of the bones) that can effect your bone health in the not-too-distant future
- Difficulty conceiving, even when you have resumed normal menses, should you want to have a baby

Roughly 12 percent of world-class cyclists experience amenorrhea. But cyclists aren't the only women with menstrual problems. Others include:
- 12 percent of collegiate swimmers
- 24 to 26 percent of competitive runners
- 19 to 44 percent of ballet dancers
- 3 to 5 percent of the general female population

Amenorrheic women who resume menses do restore some
of the bone density lost during their months of amenorrhea,
particularly if they are younger than seventeen years. But they
do not restore all of it. Your goal should be to minimize the
damages of amenorrhea by eating appropriately and taking the
proper steps to regain your menstrual periods. Remember, food
is fuel, healthful and health-giving, not a fattening enemy.

● **RESOLVING AMENORRHEA**—The possible changes required
to resume menses include:
- Training 5 to 15 percent less, for instance, 50 minutes instead
  of an hour
- Consuming 10 percent more calories each week until you
  ingest an appropriate amount given your activity level. For
  example, if you have been eating 1,500 calories a day, eat 150
  more calories per day for a total of 1,650 total calories per
  day during the first week; eat 150 calories more per day for a
  total of 1,800 calories per day during the second week; 1,950
  calories per day during the third week, and so on.
- Choosing more protein- and calcium-rich foods, such as
  (Greek-style) yogurt
- Gaining a few pounds
  Some amenorrheic cyclists have resumed menses with just
reduced exercise and no weight gain. An injured cyclist who
totally stops training might resume menses within two months.
Others resume menstruating after rebuilding and restoring five
pounds (or less) of health. And despite what you may think,
this small amount of weight gain tends to include muscle-
weight and does not result in your "getting fat."

● STEPS TO RESOLVE EATING DISORDERS

If you are spending too much time obsessing about food, weight, and exercise, seek help and information by contacting:

- National Eating Disorders Association
  (information and referral network)
  www.NationalEatingDisorders.org

- American Dietetic Association
  (referral network)
  www.eatright.org

- Sports Nutrition group of the American Dietetic Association
  (referral network) www.SCANdpg.org

- Something Fishy Website on Eating Disorders
  (information and referral network)
  www.something-fishy.org

- Gürze Books
  (recommended self-help books)
  www.bulimia.com

If you suspect your training partner or friend is struggling with food issues, speak up! Anorexia and bulimia are self-destructive eating behaviors that may signal underlying depression and can be life-threatening. Here are some helpful tips:

- Approach the person gently but be persistent. Say that you are worried about her health. She, too, may be concerned about her loss of concentration, light-headedness, or chronic fatigue. These health changes are more likely to be a stepping stone to accepting help, since the person clings to food and exercise for feelings of control and stability.
- Don't discuss weight or eating habits. Address the fundamental problems of life. Focus on unhappiness as the reason for seeking help. Point out how anxious, tired, and/or irritable the person has been lately. Emphasize that she doesn't have to be that way.
- Post a list of resources (with tear-off websites at the bottom) where the person will see it (see resources listed above).

Remember that you are not responsible and can only try to help. Your power comes from using community resources and health professionals, such as a counselor, nutritionist, or eating disorders clinic.

If you have stopped menstruating and believe that poor eating may be part of the problem, see the helpful tips below. You should also consider getting a nutrition checkup with a registered dietitian who specializes in sports nutrition. Refer to to page 168 for more resources.

The following tips may help you resume menses or at least rule out nutrition-related factors.

1. Throw away the bathroom scale. Rather than striving to achieve a certain number on the scale, let your body weigh what it weighs. Focus on how healthy you feel and how well you perform, rather than on the number you weigh.

2. If you have weight to lose, don't crash-diet but rather slightly cut back on your food intake by cutting out only 100 to 200 calories. Severe dieters commonly lose their menstrual periods, suggesting that amenorrhea is an adaptation to the calorie deficit produced either by low calorie intake alone or by increased energy expenditure via exercise. In particular, rapid weight loss may predispose you to amenorrhea. By following a healthy reducing program, such as outlined in chapter 16, you'll not only have greater success with long-term weight loss, but also have enough energy to enjoy biking.

3. If you are at an appropriate weight, practice eating as you did as a child: Eat when you are hungry, stop when you are content. Don't stop eating just because you think you should. If you are always hungry and are constantly obsessing about food, you are undoubtedly trying to eat too few calories. Chapter 15 can help you determine an appropriate calorie intake and eating schedule that may differ from your current routine, particularly if you yo-yo between starving and bingeing.

4. Eat adequate protein. Research has suggested that amenorrheic athletes tend to eat less protein than their regularly menstruating counterparts. In one study, 82 percent of the amenorrheic women ate less than the recommended dietary allowance for protein. Vegetarians, in particular, need to be sure to consume adequate protein (see chapter 6).

5. *Eat at least 20 percent of your calories from fat.*
Amenorrheic cyclists commonly are afraid of eating fat. They
think that if they eat fat, they'll get fat. Although excess calories from fat are easily fattening, some fat (20 to 30 percent of
total calories) is an appropriate part of a healthy sports diet.
For most active people, this translates into about 40 to 60 or
more grams of fat per day. Clearly, this differs from a no-fat diet
and allows lean meats, peanut butter, nuts, olive oil, and other
wholesome foods and healthful fats that balance a sports diet
(see chapter 7).

6. *Maintain a calcium-rich diet.* You should choose a high-cal-
cium diet to help maintain bone density. Because you build
peak bone density in your teens and early adult years, your
goal is to protect against future problems with osteoporosis by
eating calcium-rich foods today. As mentioned in chapter 1, a
safe target is at least 1,000 milligrams of calcium per day if you
are between nineteen and fifty years old, and 1,200 to 1,300
milligrams of calcium per day if you are an amenorrheic or
post-menopausal woman. This is the equivalent to including a
serving of milk, yogurt, and other dairy or calcium-rich foods
at each meal in the day.

Chapter 1 provides guidelines for getting an optimal
amount of calcium. Although you may cringe at the thought of
spending so many calories on dairy foods, remember that milk
is not an "optional fluid" but rather a wholesome food that
contains many important nutrients. Some research also suggests women who consume three or more glasses of milk or
yogurt per day tend to be leaner than those who do not consume as much dairy.

Calcium is only one factor that affects bone density. There
is a genetic factor to osteoporosis; if your mother or grand-
mother has/had osteoporosis, you are more likely to inherit the
condition. Other factors that contribute to your risk for osteoporosis include being too thin with too little muscle tugging on
bones to keep them strong, doing inadequate muscle-building
exercise, and having low levels of estrogen. Lack of weight-
bearing exercise (that stimulates bone density) among cyclists
can also contribute to lower bone density.

• SUMMARY—

- Due to the prevailing myths that thinness contributes to both better performance and happiness, some cyclists consider food to be a fattening enemy rather than a friendly fuel.
- Cyclists who strive to be abnormally thin commonly pay a high price: eating disorders, poor nutrition, poorly fueled muscles, amenorrhea (in women), stress fractures and other injuries, to say nothing of reduced stamina, endurance, and performance.
- Women are supposed to have more body fat than men, yet often they target unnaturally low weights.
- Amenorrheic athletes often strive to maintain an unhealthy low weight and restrict calories. The changes that may be required to resume menses include eating more calories, reducing training, and restoring wasted muscle.
- Rather than striving to achieve a certain number on the scale, let your body weigh what it weighs. Focus on how healthy you feel and how well you perform, rather than on the number you weigh.
- Remember, food is fuel and hunger is your body's request for fuel. Eat when you are hungry and stop when you are satisfied. If you are always hungry and are constantly thinking about food, you are undoubtedly trying to eat too few calories.

Words of wisdom from other cyclists... ━━━━━━━━━━━━━━━━

"When it comes to diet and weight management, I think it's psychologically difficult for female athletes to eat as much as we need to. I think there's something in our brains that tells us that eating is bad."
Tracie Timothy, Salt Lake City, UT

"To lose weight, I used to hold back on eating, then go out and push myself on the bike. Afterward, I'd reward myself with a huge meal. Now, I eat before and during the ride to fuel the ride, and I don't deal with hunger afterwards. I have lost weight and I ride stronger."
Rich Lesnik, San Francisco, CA

"I was your typical female endurance cyclist concerned about having low body weight but suffering because I was tired all the time, lacked power in races, and didn't recover properly. I would graze constantly after long rides on nothing substantial—a handful of cereal, nibbles on loose chocolates, coffees, etc.—but did not re-fuel properly with a decent meal. I look back on how poorly I ate and wonder how I ever managed it."
Karen Sawyer, Hindmarsh, Australia

How to Gain Weight Healthfully

IF YOU ARE AMONG THE MINORITY OF CYCLISTS WHO STRUGGLE WITH being too thin, food may seem a medicine, meals a burden, and the expense of food budget-breaking. Through discipline and diet, you can change your physique to a certain extent, but first, you must have a clear picture of your genetic blueprint and a realistic goal:

• What do other people in your family look like?
• Was your mother or father very slim at your age?
• When did she or he gain weight?
• What does she or he look like now?

If, at your age, a parent was similarly thin, you probably are genetically predisposed to being thin and may have trouble adding pounds. Some people are simply "hard gainers." For example, in an overfeeding study on identical twins, some pairs of twins gained more weight than others, despite the fact that everyone overate by an equal amount—1,000 extra calories per day (Bouchard 1991). In another study, some subjects who theoretically should have gained eleven pounds during a month-long overfeeding study gained an average of only six pounds. Why the difference? Perhaps the "hard gainers" fidgeted more than others; fidgeting can burn an extra 300 to 700 calories per day! In comparison, "easy gainers" tend to enjoy sitting calmly (Levine et al. 2000).

● **SIX RULES FOR GAINING WEIGHT**—If you are a hard gainer, you can try to fidget less (unlikely!) and consume more calories than you expend. Adding muscle-building exercise such as weightlifting helps convert the extra calories into muscle rather than fat.

We encourage underweight cyclists to consume an additional 500 to 1,000 calories per day. If you are committed to the weight-gain process, you can expect to gain one-half to one pound per week, perhaps more depending on your age. For example, high school and collegiate cyclists may bulk-up more easily than the fully mature 35-year-old who is genetically skinny.

The trick to successful weight gain is to pay careful attention to these six important rules:

1. Eat consistently. Have three hearty meals plus one or two snacks daily. Do not skip meals. You may not feel hungry for lunch if you have eaten a big breakfast, but you should eat regardless. Otherwise, you will miss out on important calories you need to accomplish your goal.

2. Eat larger portions. Some people think they need to buy expensive weight-gain powders. Not true. Standard food works fine. The only reason commercial powders "work" is because they provide additional calories. If you drink the recommended three glasses per day of a 300-calorie weight-gain shake, you will consume an extra 900 calories and likely achieve the desired results. But you could less expensively consume those extra calories by eating more of readily available foods, such as:
• A bigger bowl of cereal
• A larger piece of fruit
• An extra sandwich for lunch or a large sub sandwich
• Two potatoes or two rolls at dinner instead of one
• A taller glass of milk or juice

3. Select higher-calorie foods but not higher-fat foods. Excess fat calories easily convert into body fat that fattens you up rather than bulks up your muscles. The best bet for extra calories is to choose carbohydrate-rich foods that have more calories than an equally enjoyable counterpart. For instance, an eight-ounce (240-milliliter) glass of cranberry juice has 170 calories whereas the same amount of grapefruit juice has only 100 calories. Extra carbohydrates will give you the energy you need to do muscle-building exercise. By reading food labels, you can make the best choices. See *How to Boost Your Calories* on page 174.

HOW TO BOOST YOUR CALORIES

To consume more calories, choose foods and beverages that contain more calories per serving such as those suggested here. Calorie information is for a one-cup (240-milliliter) serving unless otherwise noted.

Choose more:	Calories	Instead of:	Calories
Cranberry juice	170	Orange juice	110
Grape juice	160	Grapefruit juice	100
Banana, 1 large	170	Apple, 1 large	130
Granola	380	Bran flakes	120
Grape-Nuts	410	Cheerios	90
Corn	140	Green beans	40
Carrots	45	Zucchini	30
Split pea soup	130	Vegetable soup	80
Baked beans	260	Rice	190
Chocolate low-fat milk (1%)	160	Low-fat milk (1%)	100

4. Drink extra juice and low-fat milk. Beverages are a simple way to increase caloric intake. Instead of drinking primarily water, quench your thirst with calorie-containing fluids. One high school athlete, a client of Nancy's, gained 13 pounds over the summer by simply adding six glasses of cranberry-apple juice (about 1,000 calories) to his standard daily diet. Extra juices are a great source of calories and fluids as well as carbohydrates to keep muscles well fueled and ready to ride.

5. Do strength training (such as weightlifting and push-ups). Also called resistance training, this type of exercise stimulates muscular development, so that you bulk up instead of fatten up. Note that extra exercise, not extra protein, is the key to muscular development. If you are concerned the extra exercise will result in weight loss rather than weight gain, remember that exercise tends to stimulate the appetite. Yes, a hard ride or training session may temporarily "kill" your appetite right after the workout because your body temperature is elevated, but within a few hours when you have cooled down, you will be plenty hungry. The more you exercise, the more you will want to eat—be sure to make the time to do so.

6. Be patient. If you are in high school or college and don't easily bulk up this year, you may do so more easily as you get older. Bodies change with age! Know that you can be a strong rider by being well fueled and well trained. Your skinny legs may hurt your self-esteem more than your athletic ability.

● SUMMARY—

- You can change your physique to a certain extent, but first, have a clear picture of your genetic blueprint and a realistic goal. You may be genetically predisposed to be thin—a "hard gainer."

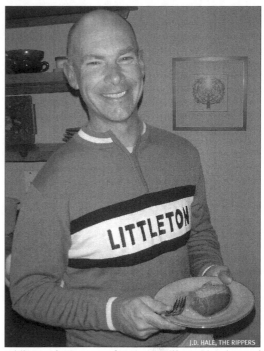

J.D. HALE, THE RIPPERS

While you don't want to fatten yourself up with cakes and pies, enjoying some dessert in moderation can fit into your sports diet.

- The bottom line for gaining weight is to consistently consume daily an additional 500 to 1,000 calories that you do not burn off. You can do that by eating larger portions, selecting higher-calorie foods but not higher-fat foods, drinking extra juice and low-fat milk, and lifting weights.
- Weight-gain powders are not necessary; you can gain weight healthfully and easily with ordinary supermarket foods.
- Just like losing weight, gaining weight takes time, patience, and perseverance.

Words of wisdom from other cyclists... ━━━━━━━

"We rode from Alaska to Argentina. There were days we felt we couldn't eat enough. One night we ate three dinners. In Peru, we walked into town and had a good dinner. Afterward, we passed another restaurant, could smell chicken roasting, and enjoyed a second dinner. Our third dinner was provided by our generous (and unsuspecting) hosts. Those were wonderful days when we were able to eat constantly and convert those calories to miles and miles."

Greg and June Siple, Missoula, MT

To find a sports nutritionist:

American Dietetic Association
Tel.: (800) 877-1600
www.eatright.org
 (click on Find a Nutrition Professional)
www.SCANdpg.org
 (to find a sports nutritionist)

Nutrition books:

*Nutrition Counseling and
Education Services*
www.ncescatalog.com

Gürze Books
www.bulimia.com

Human Kinetics
www.humankinetics.com

Cycling organizations:

Adventure Cycling Association
Tel.: (800) 755-2453 (toll-free)
www.adventurecycling.org

Adventure Cycling's mission is to inspire people of all ages to travel by bicycle. They organize tours, run instructional and leadership programs, and provide information and inspiration for cyclists. Their National Bicycle Route Network encompasses more than 40,700 miles of roads perfectly suited for cycling. Their *Adventure Cyclist* magazine is published nine times a year. Check out the Cyclosource Online Store for maps, gear, books and more.

League of American Bicyclists
Tel.: (202) 822-1333
www.bikeleague.org

Through advocacy and education, LAB works to promote safe and accessible bicycling for fun, fitness, and transportation.

Randonneurs USA
www.rusa.org

RUSA provides resources and information for non-competitive, long-distance, unsupported endurance cycling (randonneuring).

UltraMarathon Cycling Association
www.ultracycling.com

UMCA promotes the sport of long-distance and ultra-distance bicycling. *UltraCycling* magazine provides information and support for the endurance cyclist.

USA Cycling
www.usacycling.org

USA Cycling promotes and governs the sport of competitive bicycle racing and assists with athlete development.

Sports and sports nutrition:

Nancy Clark, MS, RD
www.nancyclarkrd.com
Links to nutrition articles and other nutrition sources; information on teaching materials.

Australian Institute of Sport
www.ausport.gov.au/ais
Comprehensive information on physical fitness and nutrition.

Gatorade Sports Science Institute
www.gssiweb.com

FitDay.com
www.FitDay.com
This site allows you to track and assess your food intake.

Health and nutrition:

*International Food Information
Council Foundation*
http://www.foodinsight.org
This site features information on food safety and nutrition.

Medical information
www.WedMD.com
Offers both medical and nutrition information.

*U.S. Department of Health and
Human Services*
www.healthfinder.gov
Provides information and lists organizations that produce reliable information.

Eating disorders:

National Eating Disorders Association
www.NationalEatingDisorders.org
Information, resources, and links for
resolving eating disorders.

*Something Fishy Website
on Eating Disorders*
www.something-fishy.org
Offers extensive resources and referrals
for eating disorders.

Recommended reading:

Benardot, Dan. *Advanced Sports
Nutrition.* Human Kinetics, 2006.

Clark, Nancy. *Nancy Clark's Sports
Nutrition Guidebook*, Fourth
Edition. Human Kinetics, 2008.

Colberg, Sheri. *Diabetic Athlete's
Handbook.* Human Kinetics, 2009.

Duyff, Roberta. *The American Dietetic
Association's Complete Food and
Nutrition Guide.* Chronimed
Publishing, 2006.

Freedman, Rita. *BodyLove: Learning to
Like Our Looks and Ourselves.*
Gürze Books, 2002.

Heffner, M. *The Anorexia Workbook:
How to accept yourself, heal your
suffering & reclaim your life.* 2004.

Larsen-Meyer, Enette. *Vegetarian Sports
Nutrition.* Human Kinetics, 2007.

LoBue, Andrea, and Marsea Marcus.
*The Don't Diet, Live-It! Workbook:
Healing Food, Weight & Body Issues.*
Gürze Books, 1999.

McCabe, Randi, and Traci McFarlane.
The Overcoming Bulimia Workbook.
Gürze Books, 2003.

Powers, P. and R. Thompson.
*The Exercise Balance: What's Too
Much, Too Litte, Just Right.* 2008.

Satter, Ellyn. *Secrets of Feeding a Healthy
Family.* Kelcy Press, 2008.

Siegel, Michelle, Judith Brisman, and
Margot Weinshel. *Surviving an
Eating Disorder: Perspectives and
Strategies for Families and Friends.*
HarperCollins, 2009.

Textbooks for coaches and professionals:

Manore M, N Meyer & J Thompson.
*Sport Nutrition for Health and
Performance.* Human Kinetics, 2009.

Wiliams, M. *Nutrition for Health, Fitness
& Sport.* McGraw-Hill, 2009.

SELECTED REFERENCES

Ainsworth, B., W. Haskell, M. Whitt, M. Irwin, et al. 2000. Compendium of physical activities: An update of activity codes and MET intensities. *Med Sci Sports Exerc* 32 (suppl):S498-S516.

American Dietetic Association, American College of Sports Medicine, and Dietitians of Canada. 2009. Joint Position Statement: Nutrition and Athletic Performance. *Med Sci Sports Exerc* 41 (3):709-31.

American College of Sports Medicine. 2007. Position Stand: The Female Athlete Triad. *Med Sci Sports Exerc.* 39 (10):1867-1882.

American College of Sports Medicine. 2007. Position Stand: Exercise and Fluid Replacement. *Med Sci Sports Exerc.* 39 (2):377-90.

American College of Sports Medicine. 2001. Position Stand: Appropriate Intervention Strategies for Weight Loss and Prevention of Weight Regain for Adults. *Med Sci Sports Exerc* 12:2145-56.

Armstrong, L. 2002. Caffeine, body fluid-electrolyte balance, and exercise performance. Int J Sports Nutr and Exerc Metab 12:189-206.

Armstrong, L., A. Pumerantz, M. Roti, et al. 2005. Fluid, electrolyte, and renal indices of hydration during 11 days of controlled caffeine consumption. *Int J Sport Nutr Exerc Metab* 15:252-265.

Atkinson, G., R. Davison, A. Jeukendrup, and L. Passfield. 2003. Science and cycling: current knowledge and future directions for research. J Sports Sci 21 (9):767-787.

Beelen M, Berghuis J, Bonaparte B, Ballak SB, Jeukendrup AE, van Loon LJ. 2009. Carbohydrate mouth rinsing in the fed state: lack of enhancement of time-trial performance. *Int J Sport Nutr Exerc Metab* 19 (4):400-9.

Berardi, J., T. Price, E. Noreen and P. Lemon. 2006. Postexercise muscle glycogen recovery enhanced with a carbohydrate-protein supplement. *Med Sci Sports Exerc* 38 (6):1106-1113.

Bergeron, Michael. 2008. Muscle cramps during exercise–Is it fatigue or electrolyte deficit? *Curr Sports Med Rep* 7 (4):S50-55.

Bouchard, C. 1991. Heredity and the path to overweight and obesity. *Med Sci Sports Exerc* 23 (3):285-291.

Burke LM. 2010. Fueling strategies to optimize performance: training high or training low? *Scand J Med Sci Sports* 20 (suppl) 2:48-58.

Burke, L., B. Kiens, J. Ivy. 2004. Carbohydrates and fat for training and recovery. *J Sports Sci* 22 (1):15-30.

Burke, L., G. Collier, E. Broad, et al. 2003. Effect of alcohol intake on muscle glycogen storage after prolonged exercise. *J Appl Physiol* 95 (3):983-990.

Davis, J. 1995. Carbohydrates, branched-chain amino acids and endurance: the central fatigue hypothesis. *Int J Sport Nutr* 5:S29-S38.

Dawson, D., et al. 2002. Effect of C and E supplementation on biochemical and ultrastructural indices of muscle damage after a 21 km run. *Int J Sports Med* 23 (1):10-15.

Fragakis, A. 2003. The Health Professional's Guide to Popular Dietary Supplements. Chicago, IL: American Dietetic Association, pp. 45-50.

Garner, D. 1998. "The Effects of Starvation on Behavior: Implications for Dieting and Eating Disorders." *Healthy Weight Journal* 12 (5): 68–72.

Godard, M., D. Williamson, et al. 2002. Oral amino-acid provision does not affect muscle strength or size gains in older men. *Med Sci Sports Exerc* 34 (7):1126-1131.

Hargreaves, M., J. Hawley, and A. Jeukendrup. 2004. Pre-exercise carbohydrate and fat ingestion: effects on metabolism and performance. *J Sports Sci* 22 (1):31-38.

Hawley, J. 2002. Effect of increased fat availability on metabolism and exercise capacity. *Med Sci Sports Exerc* 34 (9):1485-1491.

Hickner RC, Dyck DJ, Sklar J, Hatley H, Byrd P. 2010. Effect of 28 days of creatine ingestion on muscle metabolism and performance of a simulated cycling road race. *J Int Soc Sports Nutr* 7 (7):26.

Jentjens, R.L., K. Underwood, J. Achten, K. Currell, C.H. Mann, and A.E. Jeukendrup. 2006. Exogenous carbohydrate oxidation rates are elevated after combined ingestion of glucose and fructose during exercise in the heat. *J Appl Physiol* 100 (3):807-816.

Jentjens, R., L. Van Loon, C. Mann, A. Wagenmakers, and A. Jeukendrup. 2001. Addition of protein and amino acids to carbohydrates does not enhance post-exercise muscle glycogen synthesis. *J Appl Physiol* 91:839-846.

Jeukendrup AE. 2010. Carbohydrate and exercise performance: the role of multiple transportable carbohydrates. *Curr Opin Clin Nutr Metab Care* 13 (4):452-7.

Levine, J., S. Schleusner, and M. Jensen. 2000. Energy expenditure of nonexercise activity. *Am J Clin Nutr* 72 (6):1451-1454.

McManus, K., L. Antinoro, and F. Sacks. 2001. A randomized controlled trial of a moderate-fat, low-energy diet compared with a low-fat, low-energy diet for weight loss in overweight adults. *Int J Obes Metab Disord* 25 (10):1503-1511.

Nieman, D., et al. 2002. Influence of vitamin C supplementation on oxidative and immune changes after an ultramarathon. *J Appl Physiol* 92 (5):1070-1077.

Pendergast, D., J. Leddy, and J. Veentkatraman. 2002. A perspective on fat intake in athletes. *J Am Coll Nutr* 19 (3):345-50.

Schabort, E., A. Bosch, et al. 1999. The effect of a preexercise meal on time to fatigue during prolonged cycling exercise. *Med Sci Sports Exerc* 31 (3):464-471.

Schwenk, T. and C. Costley. 2002. When food becomes a drug: nonanabolic nutritional supplement use in athletes. *Am J Sports Med* 30 :907-916.

Sherman, W., G. Brodowicz, D. Wright, et al. 1989. Effects of 4 h preexercise carbo-hydrate feedings on cycling performance. *Med Sci Sports Exerc* 21 (5):598-604.

Sims ST, van Vliet L, Cotter J, Rehrer N. 2007. Sodium loading aids fluid balance and reduces physiological strain of trained men exercising in the heat. *Med Sci Sports Exerc* 39 (1):123-130.

Stroebele N, de Castro JM, Stuht J, Catenacci V, Wyatt HR, Hill JO. 2009. A small-changes approach reduces energy intake in free-living humans. *J Am Coll Nutr* 28 (1):63-8.

Terjung, R., et al. 2000. American College of Sports Medicine Roundtable. The physiological and health effects of oral creatine supplements. *Med Sci Sports Exerc* 32 (3):706-717.

Wee, S., C. Williams, S. Gray, and J. Horabin. 1999. Influence of low and high glycemic index meals on endurance running capacity. *Med Sci Sports Exerc* 31 (3):393-399.

Willis K, N Peterson, E. Larson-Meyer. 2008. Should we be concerned about the vitamin D status of athletes? *Int'l J Sports Nutr* 18:204-226.

Ziegenfuss T, J Landie, R Lemieux. 2010. Protein for sports-new data and new recommendations. *Strength and Conditioning J* 31 (1): 2010.

sources of, 5 (table), 10 (table), 40,
  87 (chart)
Calories: 144-151
  counting, 144-145
  daily budgeting of, 17, 145-148
  expenditure during exercise,
    145 (table), 150 (table)
  estimating need for, 146-147
  for weight gain, 173-175
  for weight reduction, 147, 152-161
Cancer, 6
Candy, 89
Carbohydrate-loading, 2-22, 54, 57, 92,
  128-137, 132 (table)
Carbohydrates: 50-57
  amount to eat, 4, 50, 93
  before cycling, 101 (table), 55, 56
  cravings. See Food Cravings
  cyclists need for, 50-51, 57, 61, 90-102
  during cycling, 51 (table), 4, 47, 55, 94
  quick versus slow digestion of, 94
  not fattening, 4, 52, 105-113
  for recovery, 117-121, 118-119 (table)
  refined, 54
  sources of, 4, 6, 27, 33-36, 50,
    51 (table), 54, 56-57, 101 (table),
    119 (table), 139-142
  stored, 46, 50, 92
Cereals: See Breakfast cereals
Cheese:
  as calcium source, 10 (table)
  fat in, 68
  as protein source, 60 (table)
Chicken:
  cooking tips for, 65
  nutritional value of, 65
  as protein source, 60 (table)
Cholesterol, dietary, 2, 62, 65
Coffee, 20-21, 43, 45, 86, 136
  See also Caffeine
Commercial sports foods, 84-91
Complete proteins, 62
Cramping:
  in muscles, 82
  in stomach. See Gastrointestinal
    problems
Crash diets, 154-155, 161 (quote), 169
Cravings. See Food cravings

Creatine, 45-46
Dehydration:
  effect on health and performance,
    74-75, 99
  prevention of, 74-75, 81, 82, 103-105,
    138-139
  See also Fluids; Sweating; Sweat rate;
    Water
Depression, 48
Diarrhea. See GI problems
Diet:
  analysis, 3 (table), 42
  balance and variety in, 1, 2-3,
    4 (table), 11, 13, 42, 130
  daily training, 130
  guidelines for healthy, 2-3
  high-protein, 52-58
  low-fat, 69-73
  moderation in, 11, 13
  vegetarian. See Vegetarian diet
  for weight gain, 172, 175
  for weight reduction, 52-59, 152-161
Dietary Guidelines for Americans, 2-3
Dietitian:
  finding, 11, 46, 176
Digestion:
  of pre-exercise meals, 92, 95-96, 102,
    130-131
Dining out. See Restaurant meals
Dinner: 22-23, 31-38
  as dining-out meal, 24
  suggestions for, 31, 56, 142
Dressings for salads. See Salad dressing
Drinking, programmed. See Fluids
Eating:
  after riding, 114-127, 149, 156
  before riding, 55, 56, 92-102, 130-131,
    156-157
  during rides, 57 (quote), 95, 98, 103-113
  on a schedule, 112 (quote), 145-149,
    155-157
  See also Carbohydrates; Diet;
    Digestion; Fast foods; Fluids;
    Pre-ride foods; Recovery Foods;
    Snacking
Eating disorders, 71-72, 162-171
  resources for, 176-177
Eggs, 64 (table), 65 (table)

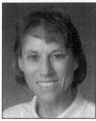

Nancy Clark, MS, RD, CSSD, an internationally respected board certified specialist in sports dietetics (CSSD), counsels both competitive athletes and casual exercisers at her private practice in the Boston area. Her clients include the spectrum from novice cyclists to Olympic hopefuls.

Clark completed her undergraduate degree in nutrition from Simmons College in Boston, her dietetic internship at Massachusetts General Hospital, and her graduate degree in nutrition with a focus on exercise physiology from Boston University. She is a Fellow of the American Dietetic Association and the American College of Sports Medicine.

She is author of the best seller *Nancy Clark's Sports Nutrition Guidebook*, as well as her *Food Guide for Marathoners: Tips for Everyday Champions, Food Guide for New Runners: Getting It Right From the Start,* and co-author of *Food Guide for Soccer: Tips and Recipes From the Pros.*

A regular contributor for *Adventure Cyclist* magazine, Clark also writes a monthly nutrition column called "The Athletes' Kitchen," which appears regularly in over 150 sports and health publications and websites.

A regular bike commuter for over 30 years, Clark has bicycled across America as a tour leader for Adventure Cycling Association, lead several other bike tours, and, as a runner, completed several marathons. She lives in the Boston area with her husband and two children.

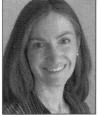

Jenny Hegmann, MS, RD, is a registered dietitian specializing in sports nutrition, wellness, and weight management. She has presented sports nutrition seminars for local cycling clubs and has written articles for print and web. She is a contributor for *UltraCycling* magazine.

Hegmann completed her undergraduate degree in dietetics from Idaho State University, her dietetic internship at Massachusetts General Hospital, and her graduate degree in human nutrition and metabolism from Boston University. She is a member of the American Dietetic Association and its affiliate, Sports, Cardiovascular, and Wellness Nutritionists.

A serious cyclist for over 20 years, Hegmann has participated in randonnées, fitness rides, and races. She is a member of the Northeast Bicycle Club and faithfully bike commutes. Hegmann is equally passionate about food and cooking and when not on her bike, can be found in her kitchen dishing up healthy feasts for family and friends. She lives and works near Boston.

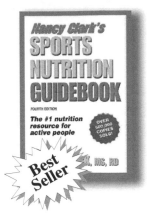
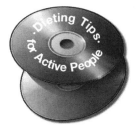
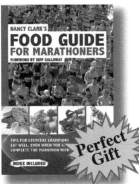